TABLE OF CONTENTS

Top 20 Test Taking Tips

1. Carefully follow all the test registration procedures
2. Know the test directions, duration, topics, question types, how many questions
3. Setup a flexible study schedule at least 3-4 weeks before test day
4. Study during the time of day you are most alert, relaxed, and stress free
5. Maximize your learning style; visual learner use visual study aids, auditory learner use auditory study aids
6. Focus on your weakest knowledge base
7. Find a study partner to review with and help clarify questions
8. Practice, practice, practice
9. Get a good night's sleep; don't try to cram the night before the test
10. Eat a well balanced meal
11. Know the exact physical location of the testing site; drive the route to the site prior to test day
12. Bring a set of ear plugs; the testing center could be noisy
13. Wear comfortable, loose fitting, layered clothing to the testing center; prepare for it to be either cold or hot during the test
14. Bring at least 2 current forms of ID to the testing center
15. Arrive to the test early; be prepared to wait and be patient
16. Eliminate the obviously wrong answer choices, then guess the first remaining choice
17. Pace yourself; don't rush, but keep working and move on if you get stuck
18. Maintain a positive attitude even if the test is going poorly
19. Keep your first answer unless you are positive it is wrong
20. Check your work, don't make a careless mistake

The Antepartal Period

Normal Pregnancy

Amenorrhea

Amenorrhea, absence of menstruation, is one of the first signs of pregnancy. Most women menstruate on a 28-day cycle with ovulation occurring at about day 14 of the cycle. The ovum remains fertile for 12 to 24 hours. For conception to occur, intercourse must take place within 5 to 6 days before and/or the day of ovulation. Sperm remain most fertile in the female reproductive tract for 24 hours. Fertilization (conception) usually takes place in the fallopian tube, and during the first 14 days (pre-embryonic stage), cell division and cell multiplication occur, forming an inner layer (blastocyst) and outer layer (trophoblast). If fertilization of the egg does not occur, the uterine lining begins to shed and menstruation occurs on about day 23. However, if the trophoblast attaches to the endometrium of the uterus (implantation), usually 7 to 10 days after fertilization, the uterine lining thickens and the trophoblast cells grow into the lining. The placenta forms and hormonal changes associated with pregnancy prevent menstruation.

Pregnancy Symptoms

Nausea and vomiting
Human chorionic gonadotropin (hCG) levels increase, and carbohydrate metabolism changes, resulting in nausea, especially in the morning. This "morning sickness" (which actually can occur at any time during the day) usually occurs 6 weeks after the last menstrual period and lasts for 6 to 12 weeks, although it may be prolonged in some women.

Fatigue
During the first trimester, the body goes through many changes as the placenta forms and the embryo grows into the fetus, causing exhaustion that is not relieved by sleeping or rest. The mother should rest as much as possible, modifying activities. Symptoms subside by the second trimester.

Urinary frequency
The growing uterus presses on the bladder, causing frequent urge to urinate, and increased vascularization increases volume of urinary output. Symptoms recede as the uterus rises into the abdomen during the second trimester but return when the uterus descends again into the pelvic area during the third trimester.

Breast changes
Breast changes (growth, engorgement, tenderness, prominent veins, stretch marks, itching) often begin to occur even before the first missed period. Hormone changes promote growth of the ductal system to prepare the breasts for milk production. Breasts usually grow about a cup size. At 6 to 8 weeks, the nipples begin to enlarge and Montgomery tubercles (bumps around the areola) become more obvious. Discomfort usually recedes after the first trimester. Support bra may help relieve discomfort.

Quickening

Movement of the fetus is usually detected at 18 to 20 weeks after the last menstrual period (LMP) in a primigravida or 16 weeks in a multigravida. Quickening is often described as a "fluttering" within the abdomen, felt when the fetus moves.

Pregnancy tests

Pregnancy should be verified by a positive pregnancy test:
- Urine tests: All tests measure human chorionic gonadotropin (hCG). Laboratory tests, such as hemagglutination-inhibition test and latex agglutination test, are 95% to 98% accurate at about 2 weeks after the first missed period. Home urine tests may detect pregnancy within a day of a missed period, but most are more accurate at 1 to 2 weeks after the missed period. False negatives are more common than false positives.
- Serum tests: These tests are more accurate than urine tests as they detect a subunit of hCG, so they may detect pregnancy even before a missed period. Additionally, monitoring of progesterone levels may help to determine if a pregnancy is viable as levels greater than 25 ng/mL suggest viability, and levels less than 5 ng/mL are inconsistent with viability.
- Ultrasound: The gestational sac can be seen transabdominally 5 to 6 weeks from the LMP and transvaginally at 3 to 4 weeks gestation

Fetal heart tones

Fetal heart tones are usually heard at about 20 weeks gestation with a fetoscope, although they may be heard much earlier with Doppler. The heartbeat has a distinctive galloping sound, more distinct as the fetus develops. Additionally, the Doppler may pick up the maternal heartbeat as well as the sound of arterial blood flow and placental blood flow (a whooshing sound). In some cases, artifacts (popping, crackling) may be heard, although using gel on the abdomen reduces artifacts. In early pregnancy, the fetal heart tones may be heard most easily above the symphysis pubis, but later finding the heart tones depends on the size and position of the fetus. Heart tones are easier to hear through the fetus's back, below the shoulder, so palpating the fetus to ascertain position, placing the fetoscope firmly against the skin, and moving the fetoscope slowly can help to locate heart tones. Auscultation should be done between contractions.

Fundal height during pregnancy

The uterine fundus (curvature at the top) can be palpated above the symphysis pubis by about 10 to 12 weeks gestation, and fundal height can be used to estimate duration of gestation and growth of the fetus. Starting at about week 16 gestation and lasting until week 36, the fundal height (from top of symphysis pubis to top of fundus) measured in centimeters usually equals the weeks of gestation, so 18 cm is consistent with 18 weeks gestation in a pregnancy with a normal single fetus. At 20 weeks (20 cm), the fundus is usually at the umbilicus. After 36 weeks, the fundal height may increase slowly or decrease as the head engages in preparation for delivery. If the baby is lying across the abdomen, the fundal height may be lower than expected, and a breech presentation usually results in increased fundal height. Multiple births result in a markedly increased fundal height.

Fetal ultrasound

Ultrasound is an imaging technique using high-frequency sound waves to create computer images of vessels, tissues, and organs. Newer scans include 2-dimensional Doppler readings. Fetal ultrasound can be done at about the fifth week of gestation and is commonly done at 20 weeks for all pregnant women. Ultrasound may be done transvaginally or (more commonly) transabdominally to evaluate the gestational sac and embryo/fetus, providing the most accurate measurement of gestational age.

During the first trimester, the purposes of an ultrasound are as follows:
- Estimate gestational age (accuracy ±1 to 2 weeks).
- Assess vaginal bleeding.
- Determine multiple fetuses.
- Examine for indications of birth defects of the brain/spine.

During the second trimester, the purposes of an ultrasound are as follows:
- Estimate gestational age (accuracy ±2 weeks).
- Determine size and position of placenta, fetus, and umbilical cord.
- Examine for indications of major birth defects (cardiovascular/neural tube).

During the third trimester, the purposes of an ultrasound are as follows:
- Estimate gestational age (accuracy ±2 to 3 weeks).
- Assess fetal viability.
- Determine size and position of placenta, fetus, and umbilical cord.
- Estimate volume of amniotic fluid.

Physiological changes of pregnancy

<u>Respiratory</u>
The following are the respiratory changes that occur during pregnancy:
- Airway engorgement: Swelling occurs in the lining of the respiratory tract, including the nose, throat, trachea, and bronchi, resulting in tonal changes in the voice, nasal congestion, and increased risk of respiratory infections
- Total lung capacity: Little change because ribs expand outward as the uterus raises the diaphragm by about 4 cm.
- Volumes: Expiratory reserve, residual, and functional residual volumes decrease by about 20% over the course of the pregnancy.
- Minute ventilation and tidal volume: MV increases by 50% by second trimester and TV increases 40%.
- Respiratory rate: Increases 2 to 3 per min.
- Oxygen consumption: Increases by about 20%.

Gastrointestinal

The gastrointestinal changes that occur during pregnancy are:

- Abdominal enlargement: Progressive abdominal enlargement associated with amenorrhea is characteristic of pregnancy. Little change is evident during the first trimester as the fundal height remains within the pelvis, but the abdomen enlarges as the uterus grows and fundal height moves upward. The stomach and intestines move upward and the stomach position becomes vertical rather than horizontal, increasing intragastric pressure and contributing to reflux.
- GI motility: Reduced as well as transit time in order to allow for more nutrients to be absorbed.
- Gallbladder: Dilates. Increased risk of gallstones.
- Appetite: Usually increased and women may experience cravings for specific foods.
- Lower esophageal sphincter: The lower esophageal sphincter is relaxed with increased production of progesterone, increasing reflux and resulting in frequent heartburn during pregnancy.

Integumentary

The integumentary changes that occur during pregnancy are:

- Stretch marks: Stretch marks, or striae gravidarum, may appear on the abdomen as well as on thighs, breasts, buttocks, or other parts of the body, especially if weight gain is fast or significant. Stretch marks are scarring that results from stretching of the tissue and tears in the dermis.
- Hyperpigmentation: Hormonal changes result in increased pigmentation and darkening of the area around the umbilicus, the midline of the abdomen (linea nigra), and characteristic darkening of areas of the face exposed to sun (chloasma).
- Skin lesions/change: Spider nevi (red with extensions resembling a spider web) and palmar erythema may result from increased levels of estrogen.

Metabolic and endocrine

The following are metabolic and endocrine changes that occur during pregnancy:

- BMR: Increases 15% to 20%.
- Weight gain: Average is about 27.5 pounds with about 1 pound associated with the fetus and the rest energy stores for the mother. Weight gain is about 1 pound per week over the final 20 weeks of pregnancy.
- Thyroid/Parathyroid: TB, T3, and T4 increase. TSH levels should remain relatively the same.
- PTH increases in response to increased calcium levels.
- Pituitary: FSH/LH decreases. Corticotropin and prolactin increase.
- Adrenal: Cortisol levels increase, facilitating production and storage of fat.
- Pancreas: Insulin resistance may develop. Insulin response increases, resulting in low glucose levels, although insulin resistance and gestational diabetes may develop as a result of this.

Hematological

The hematological changes that occur during pregnancy are:

- Blood volume: Plasma volume increases 40% to 50% and red blood cells by 20% to 30%, so the blood becomes more dilute in order to facilitate fetomaternal exchange of nutrients, oxygen, carbon dioxide, and metabolites, and to reduce the impact of blood loss during delivery.
- Blood components: White blood cell counts remain at the upper limits of normal with marked increase during and after delivery. Fibrinogen and clotting factors (VII, X, XII) increase to prevent excess bleeding during delivery. Platelet levels should remain stable or slightly increase.
- Hemoglobin: Decreased (10.5 to 13.5g/dL) in response to increased volume of plasma.
- Na and K: Slightly decreased.
- Ca and Mg: Calcium decreased and magnesium stable.
- Bilirubin: Decreased.

Renal/Urinary

The following are renal and urinary changes that occur during pregnancy:

- GFR and creatinine clearance: Increased by approximately 50%.
- Creatinine (serum) and urea: Decreased by approximately 25%.
- Protein (urine): Protein should not be present in the urine and may indicate complications.
- Residual urine volume: Increased as kidneys and ureters enlarge in response to relaxation of smooth muscles. Kidneys elongate, and ureters become longer.
- Bladder capacity: Increased with relaxation of smooth muscles, increasing risk of urinary tract infections, which may be asymptomatic, and pyelonephritis during pregnancy.
- Glucose (urine): Glucosuria may occur in up to 15% of women because of increased GFR and glucose reabsorption.
- Aldosterone: Increased 2 to 3 times to compensate for increased levels of sodium related to increased GFR.

Laboratory changes associated with pregnancy

The following are changes noted in lab tests during pregnancy:

- Hemoglobin:
  - Normal value - 11.7 to 15.5
  - Pregnancy value - 11.5 to 15
- Hematocrit:
  - Normal value - 38 to 44
  - Pregnancy value - 32 to 36.5
- Red blood cell count:
  - Normal value - 4.20 to 4.87
  - Pregnancy value – Unchanged
- White blood cell count:
  - Normal value - 4,500 to 11,000
  - Pregnancy value - 6,000 to 20,000 (increase often related to neutrophils)

- Serum creatinine:
  - Normal value - 0.5 to 1.1 mg/dL
  - Pregnancy value - 0.53 to 9.9 mg/dL
- Serum BUN:
  - Normal value - 8 to 21 mg/dL
  - Pregnancy value - 8 to 10 mg/dL
- Serum uric acid:
  - Normal value - 3.5 to 7.3 mg/dL
  - Pregnancy value - 2 to 5.8 mg/dL
- Creatinine clearance (urine):
  - Normal value - 75 to 115 mL/min
  - Pregnancy value - 150 to 200 mL/min
- Alkaline phosphatase (ALP):
  - Normal value - 25 to 125 U/L
  - Pregnancy value - Increase 2 to 4 times

Expanding family developmental tasks

Ambivalence to acceptance

Almost all mothers have feelings of ambivalence about the challenges of parenthood, and these feelings are normal and healthy, representing a transitional stage leading to acceptance. Areas of concern include:
- Changing body image/sexuality: Weight gain, varicose veins, growing abdomen, stretch marks, and breast changes may cause the mother to fear she is no longer attractive
- Labile moods: Hormonal and body changes can lead to rapid mood swings and emotional outbursts that may affect relationships, especially if the partner is unprepared
- Personality changes: Pregnancy often results in a tendency toward introversion, with the mother requiring more rest and personal time, and this can lead to conflicts

If the pregnancy was unintended, the mother may especially resent the pregnancy and consider abortion, leading to feelings of guilt. Many mothers are able to work through these issues and reach acceptance, especially by the third trimester when pregnancy is obvious, and people are often more solicitous and supportive. However, this is also a time of concern for the fetus.

<u>Psychosexual changes</u>
Maternal psychosexual changes vary throughout the pregnancy and afterward:
- First (1 to 13 weeks) - The first trimester can be considered a time of psychosocial crisis. The woman can experience a period of stress and anxiety, which can have a profound impact on her relationship with her partner or husband. Fears of miscarriage are not unusual. These concerns by the mother can be minimized by her partner or husband's involvement in the pregnancy, such as by accompanying the partner or wife to Lamaze classes and prenatal visits.
- Second (14 to 26 weeks) - Social myths and taboos, mostly unsubstantiated, may interfere with intimacy (particularly sexual) between the mother and her partner or husband. The mother's self-perceived body image due to an expanding abdomen and weight gain may affect her self-esteem. During this time the clinician can

intervene and counsel the couple on any restrictions associated with sexual relations.

- Third (27 to 42 weeks) - There is generally a decline in sexual interest in the mother during this period. The woman's perceived body habitus may make her feel awkward, unattractive, and uncomfortable, leading to intimacy problems between her and her partner or husband. The couple may avoid engaging in sexual intercourse fearing labor induction, bleeding, or pain. The couple feels vulnerable at this period, and it is critical that the clinician asks the couple about their intimacy in order to lead to discussion and reassurance.
- Postpartum period - Estrogen and progesterone levels drop, causing vaginal atrophy. This, combined with the vaginal and perineal trauma due to the childbirth process, may make intercourse uncomfortable for the pair. Healing lacerations or episiotomy, breastfeeding, and exhaustion, caused by the attention the new baby requires, may cause further problems with the relationship.

Paternal psychosexual changes vary with the trimesters:
- First (1 to 13 weeks) - The father may feel initial excitement or concern but then begin to feel left out as the mother gets more attention. He may not understand the mother's mood swings, and may resent changes in sexual activity. Fathers often fantasize about an older child (playing ball with a child) rather than an infant, who may not seem real at this point.
- Second (14 to 26 weeks) - While coming to terms with the pregnancy, the father may feel more connection if he goes with his partner to the doctor, listens to the fetal heartbeat, and sees the ultrasound. The father may have anxiety about his role and the expectations of the mother. If the mother is demanding of attention, he may become resentful and seek reasons to be away from home. Sexual desire may increase or decrease. The father begins to examine his relationship with his own father and to determine what type of father he wants to be.

Sibling preparation

Preparation of siblings prior to the birth of an infant can decrease anxiety and sibling rivalry by helping the children feel as though they are participants in the process and are valued. Children should be prepared for physical changes in the mother, changing family dynamics, and infant care. Formal classes may be available for children (3 to 12 years) to help them identify and express their concerns and teach them about pregnancy and child care. Booklets, books, and videos are also available. The parent/teacher may use dolls to demonstrate child care and allow the children to practice holding and caring for the baby. When possible, children should have contact with an infant, such as that of a friend or family member. Children may help to decorate the infant's room or prepare a "welcome gift," such as a drawing or toy. Children should be told who will care for them during labor and delivery and should visit the mother and infant as soon after delivery as possible.

Grandparent preparation

Grandparents may vary widely in their feelings about a pregnancy. For example, the parents of a pregnant adolescent may feel anger and despair while the parents of a mature, married adult may be thrilled. Grandparents can provide significant support and should be included in planning early in the pregnancy, but the parents should keep clear boundaries when it comes to decision-making. In some cases, there may be conflicts between the grandparents and the parents regarding religious or cultural practices. While it may be difficult to confront these issues, it's better to deal with them during the pregnancy than after delivery. The parents should state their desires and plans openly, giving their reasons. Grandparents may benefit from classes or a review of current standards and practices in relation to pregnancy, delivery, and breastfeeding.

Rest

A mother often feels fatigued and must ensure she gets adequate rest. Fatigue is especially pronounced during the first trimester, usually eases in the second, and returns in the third. Strategies to increase rest include:
- Increase nighttime sleep to 8 to 10 hours by going to bed earlier or sleeping later
- Experiment with different positions during sleep, but avoid lying on the stomach because this will be uncomfortable as the uterus grows. Using pillows to support the body may relieve discomfort
- Take rest breaks or short naps during the daytime
- Change work/social schedule by working fewer hours if possible or eliminating unnecessary meetings, activities, or social events
- Ask for help
- Exercise daily, such as walking
- Eat a healthy diet and drink ample fluids

Bathing

Because of increased perspiration and vaginal discharge, pregnant women should bathe daily and may shower or take a tub bath as desired throughout pregnancy. It may be difficult for a woman to get safely in and out of a tub during the third trimester, so she may need assistance, tub mats, and safety bars. Tub bathing is contraindicated if the woman is experiencing vaginal bleeding or the membranes have ruptured.

Dressing

Generally, clothing should be comfortable and nonconstrictive. Women excited about pregnancy often begin wearing maternity clothes earlier than women who want to hide pregnancy or feel negatively about it. Girdles are not advised unless the woman has a large pendulous abdomen, but girdles should never be constrictive around the legs as they may decrease peripheral circulation. As pregnancy progresses, women often choose clothing that is easy to get on and off.

Exercising

Moderate exercise, such as walking, should be done for 30 minutes daily. Supine exercises should be avoided during the second and third trimesters because this position decreases maternal cardiac output and uterine circulation. Aerobic exercises should be modified, and exercises that require balance (gymnastics, horseback riding, skiing) should be avoided. Generally pulse rate during exercise should not be higher than 140.

Grooming

Pregnant women often experience an increase in acne because of hormonal changes but should avoid cleansing preparations that contain salicylic acid or antiaging compounds with retinoids. Women should avoid hair dye and permanent waves because some of the chemicals are teratogenic, especially during the first trimester. Henna is a natural product that is safe. Lemon juice can be used to lighten facial hair rather than bleach products. Soy products may increase melasma because of estrogenic properties. Chemical hair removers and sunscreen products are generally safe for pregnant women. Most makeup is safe except for those that contain retinol or salicylic acid.

Traveling

If a pregnant woman is healthy with no fetal complications, travel is usually not restricted; however, long automobile trips should be avoided in favor of air or train travel. If traveling by car, the woman should get out and walk for 10 minutes at least every 2 hours. She should wear both a lap belt, positioned under the abdomen and across the upper thighs and shoulder strap positioned between the breasts. Flying is acceptable until week 36 but is contraindicated with obstetric complications, placental abnormalities, or increased risk of premature delivery.

Working

Work/employment that requires prolonged standing or demanding physical activities is associated with increased premature delivery, so work should be evaluated on an individual basis. Women should avoid working with fetotoxic hazards/chemicals and may need reassignment. In the third trimester, balance is impaired, and this may be a consideration for some jobs. One of the biggest problems associated with working is fatigue, and the woman must try to find ways to get adequate rest, such as taking regular breaks or reducing hours.

Childbirth preparation exercises

The pregnant woman can benefit from a number of specific exercises, but they should be done slowly, usually in sets of 5, being careful to avoid strain:
- Pelvic tilt - Pelvic tilt strengthens both muscles in the lower back and lower abdomen, reducing back strain. Pelvic rocking is best done in the supine position with feet flat on the floor, but it can also be done on hands and knees, standing against a wall, or sitting in a chair
- Abdominal tightening - This exercise involves pulling the abdominal muscles tight while exhaling. This exercise is most easily practiced while lying supine with feet flat on the floor
- Partial sit-ups - Partial sit-ups strengthen abdominal muscles. The woman should lie in supine position with knees flexed and feet flat on the floor, stretching arms toward the knees while lifting the head and neck
- Thigh stretching - Sitting in a cross-legged position stretches the muscles in the inner thighs, facilitating the birth process

<u>Kegel exercises</u>

Kegel exercises strengthen the pelvic floor muscles, which cross the floor of the pelvis and attach to the pubic bone and coccyx. The urethra, rectum, and vagina open through the pelvic floor muscles, which support the pelvic organs. Strengthening these muscles helps prevent stress incontinence and childbirth-related disorders, such as uterine prolapse, rectocele, and cystocele.

- Caution: Avoid holding the breath or tightening the abdominal or buttocks muscles during pelvic floor exercises
- Procedure: Tighten and squeeze the muscles about the rectum, vagina, and urethra, and try to "lift" them inside as though trying to stop from passing gas and urine. Hold. Relax. Rest a few seconds. Repeat
- Schedule: Exercises should be done at least 3 times daily. They may be done while lying down in the morning and evening and while sitting midday
  - Initially: Tighten 1 second, relax 5. Repeat 5 to 10 times
  - Later: Tighten 5 seconds or longer and relax 10. Repeat 10 times

Pregnancy nutritional needs

The nutrition of the mother has a profound effect on the developing embryo/fetus. Caloric needs vary widely depending on the mother's age, size, weight, metabolism, and general health. Energy needs of the mother usually remain stable during the first trimester but an added 300 kilocalories a day are needed during the second and third trimester for a singleton and 600 kilocalories a day for twins. Recommended dietary intake for pregnant women includes:

- A (μg/d) - 750 to 770
- C (mg/d) - 80 to 85
- D (mcg/d) - ≥ 5
- E (mg/d) - 15
- K (mcg/d) - 75 to 90
- Ca (mg/d) - 1,000 to 1,300
- P (mg/d) - 700 to 1,250

Generally, a pregnant woman requires about 60 g of protein daily (3 meat servings or equivalent) and 4 to 5 cups of milk (or equivalent). Diet should include 2 to 4 servings of fruit and 3 to 5 servings of vegetables. Simple carbohydrates (sugar, flour) should be limited and replaced by whole grains, which are high in B vitamins. Fat should constitute about 30% of total caloric intake.

Maternal malnutrition

Maternal malnutrition can have a profound effect on the developing fetus. If malnutrition occurs during the stages of cell division, cells may not divide properly, causing permanent damage. If malnutrition occurs when cells are enlarging, then correcting the nutritional deficit can reverse damage. Recommendations for maternal weight gain:

- Underweight: 28 to 40 lb
- Normal weight: 25 to 35 lb
- Overweight: 15 to 25 lb
- Obese: 15 lb

Malnourished or underweight mothers have increased perinatal losses and preterm births. Neonates often have lower Apgar score and low birth weight (less than 2,500 g). Women with eating disorders are more likely to have infants that are small for gestational age. Vitamin and mineral deficiencies can cause abnormalities in the developing fetus:

- Thiamine: Congestive heart failure, stillbirths.
- Folic acid: Megaloblastic anemia, neural tube defects.
- Vitamin D and calcium: Skeletal defects.

Infants of obese and morbidly obese women are often macrosomic (large) and may suffer fetal distress, early neonatal death, meconium aspiration, shoulder dystocia, and/or complications from cesarean birth.

Folic acid

Folate/Folic acid is necessary for synthesis of DNA and RNA and cell duplication. Folic acid deficiency causes megaloblastic anemia in which immature red blood cells enlarge rather than divide, resulting in fewer red blood cells. Because of the need for cell duplication during pregnancy, adequate folic acid is critical, especially because there is increased urinary excretion and fetal uptake. Women should receive 0.4 mg of folic acid daily and, for deficiency, 1 mg of folic acid and iron supplements (because folic acid deficiency is associated with iron deficiency anemia). Deficiency may be difficult to diagnose because folate levels fluctuate with diet. Women with inadequate folic acid intake often exhibit nausea, vomiting, lack of appetite, and low hemoglobin. Folic acid deficiency is associated with neural tube defects, such as myelomeningocele, spina bifida, and anencephaly, in the fetus.

Iron

Iron is necessary for the development of red blood cells. During pregnancy, the mother's plasma volume increases by about 50%, but red cell mass increases less, so the hematocrit drops from a normal of 38% to 47% to as low as 34% (physiologic anemia of pregnancy). Because the fetus takes iron from the mother, the mother's iron intake must compensate for this loss. Recommended daily iron supplements include:

- Hematocrit within normal range: 30 mg of elemental iron daily.
- Maternal iron deficiency anemia: 60 to 120 mg daily until hematocrit normalizes, at which point the dosage should decrease to 30 mg daily.

When hemoglobin falls below 11 g/dL, the mother is at increased risk of infection, preeclampsia, and postpartal hemorrhage with associated dangers to the fetus. If hemoglobin falls below 6 g/dL, the mother may suffer cardiac failure, and the fetus is at high risk through increased rates of miscarriage and stillbirth, low birth rate, and neonatal death.

Fetal growth and embryo development

The stage of the embryo begins 15 days after conception. During this stage, organs begin to form, and external features become evident. The fetus is most vulnerable to teratogenic agents during the time that organs are developing.

Week 3

The embryo elongates with a larger cephalic end than caudal. A long tube is developing for the brain and spinal cord and another for the GI system. The primitive tubular heart is forming outside the body cavity of the embryo. Teratogens may cause congenital limb absence.

Week 4

The heart beats regularly, and arm, leg, and tail buds are evident. The primordia of the eyes and ears are beginning to form. Teratogens may cause omphalocele, tracheoesophageal fistula, or hemivertebrae.

Week 5

Eyes (laterally positioned) and nasal pits are forming. The C-shaped body has a large head and tail. By the end of week 5, arm and leg buds with paddle-like hands and feet are evident. Teratogens may cause cataracts, microphthalmia, facial clefts, and/or carpal or pedal ablation.

Week 6

Arms and legs are growing and digits forming. The jaws, upper lip, palate, and ears are developing. The tail is receding. The heart has chambers and is pumping blood through the circulatory system. Teratogens may cause septal/aortic defects, cleft lip, and/or agnathia.

Week 7

The head is assuming a round shape, and eyes are moving closer together. The mouth is formed and tongue developing. Eyelids are forming. The GI and urinary tracts have separated. Fetal heartbeats are detectable. Teratogens may cause intraventricular septal defects, pulmonary stenosis, cleft palate, epicanthus, micrognathia, short head, and sexual ambiguity.

Week 8

The embryo is about 3 cm CR (crown to rump) length and resembles a human being, but the gender is not yet identifiable. Long bones are beginning to form, the heart has developed, the circulatory system is established, and muscles contract. Nose, eyes, and ears are evident. Teratogens may cause persistent atrial septal opening and shortening of digits.

9 to 12 weeks

After 8 weeks, the embryo is considered a fetus as all organs and external structures are present to some degree. After 9 weeks, the fetus has reached about 5 cm CR length, weight 14 g, with the head comprising about 50% of the total size. The neck is evident and separate from the trunk. At 12 weeks, the fetus has reached 8 cm CR length, weight 45 g, and facial features are more developed. The fetus appears human with a nose, small chin, and ears. Lip movement (sucking) may be seen, and tooth buds appear. Limbs have lengthened, and digits are well formed with arms longer and more developed than the legs. The fetus can make a fist. The urinary system has developed, and differentiated genitals appear. The fetus has spontaneous movement, and fetal heart tones are heard by Doppler.

13 to 20 weeks

At 13 weeks, the fetus has reached 9 cm CR length, weight 55 to 60 g. Growth is rapid during this period, and the gender should become evident. Eyelids have formed and can blink, and lanugo develops. The skin is transparent, so vasculature shows through. Sweat glands and fingerprints (fingers and toes) begin to develop. Bones and muscles are growing and developing, and the fetus is much more active. The fetus makes sucking movements, swallows amniotic fluid, and produces meconium. The bronchial tubes branch out, and the liver and pancreas begin to produce secretions. By week 16, the bones begin to ossify.

20 weeks
At 20 weeks, the fetus is 19 cm CR length and 435 to 465 g and is covered with lanugo with increased scalp hair. Brown fat deposits make skin more opaque, and nipples are evident. Nails, eyebrows, and eyelashes are forming. The muscles are more developed; the fetus can suck the thumb and yawn and is increasingly active. The mother feels quickening.

24 weeks
At 24 weeks, the fetus measures 28 cm CH (crown to heel) in length with weight 780 g. The lungs are developing with alveoli forming. The eyes have formed completely. The grasp and startle reflexes are obvious by the end of 24 weeks. There is little subcutaneous fat, so the skin is wrinkled and reddish in color but is completely covered with vernix caseosa. The palms and soles of the feet have thickened, and skin ridges are evident. Hair, eyebrows, and eyelashes are growing. The fetus remains active, sometimes hiccoughing and responding to sounds and activity by moving.

25 to 28 weeks
At 25 to 28 weeks, the brain and central nervous system are developing and regulating some body function. The eyelids open and close, and the lungs are developed enough to provide gas exchange. Testes begin to descend into the scrotum. By week 28, the fetus measures 35 to 38 cm CH length, weight 1,200 to 1,250 g, and may be viable if delivered prematurely but will require extended intensive care.
29 to 32 weeks: By week 32, the fetus measures 38 to 43 cm CH length, weight 2,000 g, with increased muscles and fat, so the skin is less wrinkled. The pupillary response is present. Lungs are still immature, but the central nervous system can control breathing and temperature. Bones are developed but soft. Testes may have descended.

35 to 36 weeks
By week 36, the fetus has gained more subcutaneous fat, so the skin is smoother and shedding lanugo. The brain is well developed, and lungs are almost developed. The fetus measures 42 to 48 cm CH length with weight 2,500 to 2,750 g. Nails have grown to the ends of the digits, and the hands can grasp. The fetus orients to light. If delivered, the neonate has a good chance of survival. Testes have descended to the upper scrotum for males, and the labia majora and labia minora are equal size for females.

38 to 40 weeks
By week 38, the fetus is full-term, measuring about 48 to 52 cm CH length, weight 3,000 to 3,600 g. Males tend to be slightly larger than females, but wide variations occur. The fetus is plumper with smooth skin, and lanugo remains primarily on the shoulders and upper arms with scalp hair about 1 inch in length. The head remains slightly larger than the chest, which is prominent with protruding mammary glands. Testes have fully descended or are palpable in the inguinal canals. The labia majora are well developed with labia minora smaller or covered. By this time, amniotic fluid has decreased to about 500 mL, as the fetus fills the uterus. The fetus gains protective antibodies from the mother. Vernix caseosa remains present, more obvious in skin folds and creases. The fetus usually has turned with the head pointed downward toward the birth canal. Delivery usually occurs around week 40.

IUGR

When a fetus does not fulfill his or her growth potential for any reason, the diagnosis is intrauterine growth restriction (IUGR). Prenatal ultrasound is used to diagnose IUGR, which is associated with oligohydramnios (decreased amniotic fluid) and preeclampsia (pregnancy-induced hypertension and proteinuria). IUGR is classified as symmetric or asymmetric, based on the size of the newborn's head:

- Symmetric IUGR
  - Both head and body are small (growth-restricted)
  - Occurs early in pregnancy
  - Common causes are chromosomal abnormalities and infections
- Asymmetric IUGR
  - Large head in proportion to the body; the head is spared
  - The head is normal in size for gestational age, while the body is growth-restricted
  - Occurs late in pregnancy
  - Common causes include placental insufficiency and preeclampsia

Fetal macrosomia

Fetal macrosomia, an exceptionally large fetus, poses problems for vaginal delivery because of the size of the infant. Fetal macrosomia is defined variably as greater than 90th percentile for weight according to gestational age or greater than 4,500 g. Fundal height at least 4 cm above that expected for gestational age may be an indication. Fetal macrosomia is common with infants of diabetic mothers as well as obese mothers or those who gain an excessive amount of weight during pregnancy. Complications include prolonged second stage of labor because of over-stretching of the myometrium. If the fetus is too large to descend, uterine rupture may occur. Vaginal birth often results in lacerations or extensive episiotomy. The mother has increased risk of postpartum hemorrhage. The most common complication is shoulder dystocia, sometimes resulting in permanent brachial plexus injury to the neonate. Identifying fetal macrosomia prior to labor helps to prevent complications, but ultrasound and palpation are not always reliable when estimating fetal size/weight.

Parent classes

Prepregnancy and first trimester
Classes that focus on the becoming pregnant or understanding the early stages of pregnancy often cover methods of ensuring a healthy pregnancy and preventing complications. Topics may include sexuality, nutrition, lifestyle changes, and exercise, as well as fetal development and gestational changes.

Second and third trimester
Later classes focus more on the birth process and labor as well as the postpartal period. Infant stimulation techniques, such as stroking the abdomen, rocking, and playing music, help to develop early parental bonding and skills. Topics covered may include birth choices (natural childbirth, epidural, spinal, cesarean birth), episiotomy, and circumcision, as well as discussions of safety measures, such as infant car seats and types of cribs.

Adolescent

Classes that focus on adolescent mothers help the young mothers adapt to changes in their bodies and cope with psychosocial changes, as well as preparing them for labor and delivery.

Bradley method

The Bradley method of natural childbirth is usually taught in a series of 12 weekly classes in which the pregnant woman and her partner participate. Classes are small (3 to 6 couples), and the goal is for natural childbirth without the use of drugs, cesarean birth, or episiotomy to ensure both the mother and infant are healthy. Classes begin with a focus on the woman's health, including avoiding risk factors, ensuring good nutrition, and learning to handle pain. All issues related to pregnancy, such as anatomy, physiology, fetal changes, sexual activity, and breastfeeding are discussed. The role of the father/coach and the importance of bonding exercises are stressed. The couple learns methods to help promote relaxation and control pain during all stages of labor and delivery, using breath control and deep abdominopelvic breathing. The couple also learns about the needs of the newborn and routine care.

Lamaze method

The Lamaze method encourages women to take control of their bodies and utilizes various techniques (dissociation relaxation, relaxation exercises, and breathing patterns) to alleviate discomfort and facilitate birth. Lamaze teaches that birth is a natural process that should be as free of interventions/medications as possible. Birthing practices include:
- Natural onset of labor without induction.
- Movement during labor (e.g., walking, rocking, sitting on a birth ball, taking a shower) rather than lying in bed
- Support system, including partner and a person knowledgeable about birth, such as a doula, midwife, or friend
- Only necessary medical interventions: Food and drink should not be restricted. Methods to speed labor, such as artificial rupturing of membranes, should be avoided, as well as continuous fetal heart monitoring because it restricts the mother's activities
- Avoidance of supine delivery: Upright, side lying, and hands and knees position are taught for use during different phases to speed or slow labor. Directed breathing techniques are also taught
- Skin-to-skin contact at birth and rooming-in

Kitzinger method

The Kitzinger (psychosexual) method encourages women to take an active part in the birthing process, which is viewed as very natural. Kitzinger encourages alternatives to the usual hospital birthing procedures, such as home births, birth rooms, and water births. Women learn chest breathing combined with abdominal relaxation, touch relaxation, and visualization. The Kitzinger method relies on sensory memories, using some acting techniques to help women get in touch with feelings, as well as specific movements (called "birth dance") to use during labor to reduce discomfort. In addition, the Kitzinger method includes educating the mother about pregnancy (including both physical and emotional development), fetal development, options available to her, and social and cultural aspects of birth. Women are encouraged to create a birth plan.

HypoBirthing method

The HypnoBirthing method combines natural birthing and self-hypnosis to help the mother eliminate stress and fear related to birthing. The mother is taught methods to relax the mind and body and encourage production of natural endorphins. HypnoBirthing includes teaching the mother different relaxation and breathing techniques (such as deep breathing and slow breathing), pushing techniques, and birth positions. The partner is taught to use therapeutic touch and prompts to help the mother. Additionally, HypnoBirthing includes general education about pregnancy (including early labor signs), nutrition, exercise, breastfeeding, and bonding, as well as postpartum depression. One characteristic technique is "breathing the baby down" by inhaling and then exhaling while visualizing the energy going toward the fetus while tilting the pelvis up and gently bearing down. While bearing down, the mother visualizes the vagina opening to allow passage of the fetus.

True vs. false labor

Braxton-Hicks contractions, also known as "false labor," occur during the third trimester with uterine contractions only. Uterine contractions occur throughout pregnancy but are often too mild for the woman to feel; however, as birth nears, the contractions become stronger and may be mistaken for true labor.

Braxton-Hicks:
- Remain short in duration
- Occur at irregular intervals, which do not shorten over time.
- Pain typically in lower abdomen.
- Activities (walking, taking a warm bath, resting, or drinking ample fluids) may relieve pain and lesson contractions.
- Mild analgesia may relieve discomfort.
- Cervix remains unchanged.

True labor contractions:
- Begin short in duration, but duration increases.
- Occur at regular intervals, which typically shorten over time and become more frequent.
- Pain typically is felt first in lower back and then radiates anteriorly to the abdomen.
- Activities may cause increase in pain and frequency and intensity of contractions.
- Mild analgesia usually does not provide pain relief.
- Cervical effacement and dilatation evident.

Impending labor signs

Signs of impending labor (usually weeks 38 to 42) can include:
- Lightening: As the fetal head engages and moves toward the birth canal, the fundal pressure on the diaphragm lessons, so the mother can breathe more easily, but pressure in the pelvic area increases, causing urinary frequency. The lower abdomen may protrude more than previously. Increased circulatory impairment may cause venous stasis and ankle edema, as well as increased vaginal secretions as vaginal mucous membranes become congested. Pressure on the nerves may result in leg cramps or increased pelvic and leg pain.

- Braxton-Hicks contractions: Intensity and frequency of BH contractions often increase immediately prior to onset of true labor.
- Change in energy: Mothers often experience a burst of energy and exhibit "nesting" activities, such as organizing the infant's room, preparing food, and cleaning house, usually in the week before labor starts.
- Bloody show: A mucous plug from pooled secretions forms at the opening of the cervical canal during pregnancy, and when the cervix begins to efface, this mucous plug is expelled, exposing capillary vessels that bleed. The bloody show typically appears as pink mucous as opposed to the more brownish discharge associated with manual vaginal examination of the cervix. Bloody show usually occurs within 24 to 48 hours of the onset of labor.
- Cervical changes: The cervix ripens (softens) to allow for effacement and dilation.
- GI upset: Some of the symptoms often associated with the first trimester of pregnancy may return as labor nears. These symptoms include nausea, vomiting, heartburn, and diarrhea.
- Pain: Relaxin hormone production increases markedly (10 X) during pregnancy to relax the pelvic joints and allow them to expand, but this may result in pain, especially in the lumbosacral and pelvic areas.
- Membrane rupture: Rupture of the membranes occurs in about 12% of women prior to onset of labor, which usually then occurs within 24 hours. Before rupture, the membranes typically bulge through the dilating cervix, and fluid comes in a gush, although it may come in smaller spurts in some cases. If the membranes rupture before engagement of the fetal head, the umbilical cord may prolapse with the fluid, increasing risk to the fetus, so mothers should be advised to always seek medical attention after rupture. If the mother is term and labor does not start within 24 hours of rupture, labor may be induced.
- Weight loss: Estrogen and progesterone levels cause a change in fluid balance that often results in a 1- to 3-pound loss of weight prior to onset of labor.

Onset of labor evaluation

Evaluation procedures to assess onset of labor include:
- History: Records should be reviewed and mother questioned about the onset of contractions, frequency, and duration, and whether membranes have ruptured or vaginal bleeding has occurred.
- Leopold maneuvers: Abdominal palpations are done to establish fetal position, including lie, presentation, and position. Four maneuvers include (1) determining which fetal part is at the fundus, (2) locating the fetal extremities, (3) identifying the presenting part (head, breech) of the fetus, and (4) palpating for cephalic prominence.
- Vaginal exam: Speculum exam should precede digital exam if unclear whether membranes have ruptured. Vaginal exam to check for effacement and dilation is usually delayed until after labor begins. The position of the cervix is checked: Anterior position usually indicates the fetus is descending and applying pressure.
- Fetal station: The level of the fetal presenting part is determined in relation to the ischial spines. Level with the ischial spines (indicating engagement) is designated as station 0 with levels above designated with minus (–) signs and below with plus (+) signs.

Pregnancy discomforts

Nausea and vomiting
Cause:
- **First trimester:** hCG secretion of the blastocyst and changes in carbohydrate metabolism cause nausea.
- **Second and third trimester:** Pressure of growing uterus displaces the stomach upward and the intestines laterally and downward. Gastric emptying and peristalsis slows, causing bloating and constipation. Smooth muscles relax (from elevated progesterone), resulting in gastric reflux and heartburn, which further aggravate nausea and can lead to vomiting.

Preventive measures:
- Eat small, frequent meals
- Avoid fatty, spicy foods
- Eat simple carbohydrate foods, such as saltine crackers
- Drink herbal tea with sugar or ginger ale

Medical treatment:
- Antacids: Calcium carbonate, magnesium hydroxide, or magnesium oxide
- Antihistamine/anticholinergic: Meclizine
- Antiemetics: Ondansetron, prochlorperazine, promethazine, metoclopramide, or trimethobenzamide

Heartburn
Cause: Increased progesterone combined with decreased GI motility, relaxation of the cardiac sphincter, and upward displacement of stomach from pressure of the growing uterus increase esophageal reflux.

Management:
- Eat 4 to 5 small meals rather than 3 large meals daily
- Take low-sodium antacids (NOT sodium bicarbonate)
- Avoid lying down within 2 hours of eating
- Avoid fried or spicy foods that trigger symptoms

Ankle/Foot edema
Cause: Increased sodium retention from hormonal changes, circulatory impairment to lower extremities from pressure of uterus during second and third trimesters, prolonged sitting/standing, and increased permeability of capillaries cause edema.

Management:
- Elevate feet and legs when sitting
- Avoid restrictive clothing, socks, or other bands around legs
- Exercise feet frequently while sitting
- Walk to promote increased circulation

Ptyalism
Cause: Cause is unclear for excessive salivation during first trimester.

Management:
- Use astringent mouthwashes
- Chew gum or suck on hard candy

Nasal stuffiness/Bleeding
Cause: Increased production of estrogen during first trimester causes swelling and irritation of mucous membranes.

Management:
- Use cool-air vaporizer
- Do NOT use nasal sprays/decongestants

Vaginal discharge/Monilial infection
Cause: Increased estrogen promotes hyperplasia of vaginal mucosa and increased production of mucous. Warm, moist environment promotes Candida monilial infection.

Management:
- Bathe daily.
- Wear cotton panties (NOT nylon or pantyhose).
- AVOID douching, panty liners, and tight clothing.
- Topical treatments: miconazole, butoconazole, clotrimazole, tioconazole, nystatin, or terconazole.

Leg cramps
Cause: Calcium/phosphorus imbalance occurs, increased pressure on nerves or impaired lower peripheral circulation from growing uterus, general fatigue, and pointing toes and shortening muscles may cause cramps.

Management:
- Dorsiflex feet to stretch muscles
- Modify diet to improve calcium/phosphorus balance
- Apply heat to cramping muscles
- Change position slowly

Constipation
Cause: Increased progesterone levels slow intestinal motility. Pressure on intestines from enlarging uterus, inadequate diet/fluid intake, lack of exercise, and iron supplements all slow motility.

Management:
- Increase fluids and fiber in diet
- Use stool softeners, such as DSS
- AVOID laxatives, which may increase constipation over time

Hemorrhoids
Cause: Constipation and pressure on hemorrhoidal veins from growing uterus cause veins to dilate.

Management:
- Treat constipation
- Apply ice packs
- Take sitz baths
- Apply topical ointments, such as *Preparation H* or cortisone ointment
- Apply topical anesthetic agent

Varicose veins
Cause: Venous congestion from pressure of uterus and impaired circulation, increased weight, age, and hereditary factors contribute to varicosities.

Management:
Elevate feet and legs frequently. Avoid prolonged standing, crossing legs, and wearing constrictive hosiery or clothing. Wear support hose.

Backache
Cause: Increased hormone levels cause softening of cartilage and increased lumbosacral curvature. Muscle strain, fatigue, poor body mechanics, and carrying twins contribute to backache.

Management:
- Do the pelvic-tilt exercise
- Utilize correct body mechanics. Avoid heavy lifting, reaching for things on high surfaces, and wearing high-heeled shoes
- Adjust height of work surfaces. Apply heat to lower back. Use back support in chair/bed. Begin modified exercise program, such as swimming, beginning with stretching. Stand straight and avoid slumping

Antepartal tests

APF
Alpha-fetoprotein (AFP) is a protein produced by the yolk sac for the first 6 weeks of gestation and then by the fetal liver. Cutoff levels have been established for each week of gestation, with peak levels at about week 15. The test is used primarily to detect neural tube defects (NTDs), which develop in the first trimester. AFP can be measured in amniotic fluid or maternal serum.

Triple screening
Triple screening includes serum AFP level done in the second trimester and a positive result (which may be the result of errors in the duration of gestation) is then followed by ultrasound and amniocentesis to check the amniotic AFP level. There is increased production of AFP with NTDs, as well as abdominal wall defects and congenital nephrosis, so these levels can be used for assessment. (High-quality ultrasound may also provide evidence of neural tube defects.) The accuracy of tests varies depending on the week of gestation. The most accurate results are acquired with testing during weeks 15 to 16.

CVS

Chorionic villus sampling (CVS) in which a small sample of chorionic villi is obtained from the placenta can be done within the first trimester (at least 10 weeks) to test for genetic/DNA and metabolic abnormalities, although CVS cannot detect neural tube disorders. The risk of miscarriage related to the procedure is now about the same as for amniocentesis (1:1,600); additionally, CVS can provide earlier diagnosis and fast results (within 1 day for some methods). For the procedure, an ultrasound is used to detect placental location, so the mother must drink fluids to fill the bladder. Sampling may be done transcervically with a catheter inserted through the cervix to the sampling site. Sampling may also be done transabdominally with local anesthesia and a needle inserted through the abdomen and uterine myometrium and advanced to the sampling site under ultrasound guidance.

PUBS

Percutaneous umbilical blood sampling (PUBS), also called cordocentesis, involves obtaining fetal blood from the umbilical cord in utero to diagnose hemophilia and other blood disorders, infection, and chromosomal abnormalities. During the procedure, an ultrasound is used to locate the umbilical cord and umbilical vein. A spinal needle is inserted through the abdominal wall and uterus and guided into the umbilical vein and a blood sample is aspirated. A paralytic agent, such as pancuronium bromide, is often used to prevent the fetus from moving during the procedure. The mother must avoid deep breathing during the procedure as this may interfere with puncturing the vein. While any invasive procedure increases the risk of miscarriage, the rate of miscarriage with PUBS is only about 2%.

Amniocentesis

Amniocentesis is done at 15 to 20 weeks for genetic diagnoses and at 30 to 35 weeks to determine fetal lung maturity. Ultrasound locates the placenta and fetus and identifies an area with adequate amniotic fluid. The needle is inserted carefully to avoid major structures, the fetus, and arteries. A local anesthetic may be administered before insertion of a 22-gauge spinal needle into the uterine cavity. The first drops of fluid are discarded and a syringe attached. About 15 to 20 mL of amniotic fluid are withdrawn and placed in tubes, brown-tinted to shield the fluid from light that might break down bilirubin or other pigments. Ultrasound is again used to monitor removal of the needle, and the insertion point is checked for streaming (leakage of fluid). If the mother is Rh-negative, she is given Rh immune globulin immediately unless already sensitized. The fetal heart rate is monitored. Miscarriage occurs in about 1 in 1,600. If performed at 11 to 14 weeks, there is increased risk to the fetus. Infection of the placenta (chorioamnionitis) is a rare complication.

Fetal lung maturity

Tests for fetal lung maturity are important for monitoring fetuses if there is an indication for early termination of pregnancy. Pulmonary maturity is often an important factor of neonatal survival as immaturity can result in respiratory distress syndrome (RDS). Tests of amniotic fluid include:

- Lecithin/sphingomyelin (L/S) ratio: The ratio of the phospholipids lecithin and sphingomyelin (two components of surfactant) changes during pregnancy with L/S ratio at 0.5:1 early in pregnancy, 1:1 at 30 to 32 weeks, and 2:1 at 35 weeks. At 2:1, RDS is unlikely, although this finding is not always accurate for infants of diabetic mothers (IDMs), as they may show adequate ratio but still develop RDS; these neonates must be monitored carefully. This test is not accurate if the amniotic fluid contains blood or meconium.
- Phosphatidylglycerol (PG): This phospholipid first appears in surfactant at about week 35 in IDMs with complications and week 36 in other pregnancies. Its presence is a sign of lung maturity.

Commonly, both tests are done to confirm lung maturity.

Fetal biophysical profile

The fetal biophysical profile consists of the following:

- FHR - Measures FHR and acceleration with movement as measured by the NST. The NST is done during the daytime with the woman in semi-Fowler's position with support under right hip to displace the uterus to the left. Two monitors are applied to the abdomen—an ultrasound transducer to measure FHR and a tocodynamometer to detect fetal movement. The monitoring continues for 20 to 40 minutes (time extended if fetus appears to be in sleeping cycle). Occasional decelerations are normal, but repeated decelerations correlate with increased risk of cesarean birth. The woman reports sensations of fetal movement and this is compared with recording of movement. Correlation of 50% to 90% is normal.
  - Normal (Score 2): ≥ 2 FHR accelerations of 15 BPM above baseline for ≥ 15 seconds in a 20- to 40-minute period. (Reactive)
  - Abnormal (0): 0 or 1 acceleration of FHR in 40 minutes. (Non-reactive)
- Fetal respirations: Assessed by ultrasound.
  - Normal (Score 2): ≥ 1 episode of rhythmic breathing for ≥ 30 seconds in a 30-minute period.
  - Abnormal (0): ≤ 30 seconds of rhythmic breathing in 30 minutes.
- Fetal movement: Assessed by ultrasound and tocodynamometer.
  - Normal (Score 2): ≥ 3 separate movements in 30 minutes.
  - Abnormal (0): ≤ 2 movements in 30 minutes.
- Fetal tone: Assessed by ultrasound.
  - Normal (Score 2): ≥ 2 episodes of extension and flexion of arm/leg (or opening / closing of a hand)
  - Abnormal (0): No extension/flexion

- Amniotic fluid volume: Assessed by ultrasound and amniotic fluid index. Using the umbilicus as the point of reference, the abdomen is divided into 4 quadrants and the deepest pocket in each quadrant is measured. (The sum of 4 measurements equals the amniotic fluid index [AFI].)
  - Normal (Score 2): At least 1 single vertical pocket >2 cm.
  - Abnormal (0): Largest single vertical pocket is ≤ 2 cm.

Scoring
The 5 different measurements for the biophysical profile are completed and scores (2 for normal and 0 for abnormal) are compiled and interpreted according to risk for asphyxia. Maximum score is 10:
- Score – 10. Risk of fetal asphyxia: Normal fetus with no risk. No intervention indicated.
- Score – 8. Risk of fetal asphyxia: Little/rare risk to fetus. No intervention indicated.
- Score - 8 with abnormal amniotic fluid volume. Risk of fetal asphyxia: Suspected chronic asphyxia. Increased risk of perinatal mortality ≤ 1 week (89:1,000), so birth should be induced.
- Score – 6. Risk of fetal asphyxia: Possible asphyxia. Induce birth if amniotic fluid volume abnormal, if fluid level is normal at > 36 weeks with cervix favorable, and if repeat test is ≤ 6.
- Observe and repeat tests according to protocol if repeat test is > 6.
- Score – 4. Risk of fetal asphyxia: Probable asphyxia. Repeat test the same day to verify scores and induce birth if score ≤ 6.
- Score – 2. Risk of fetal asphyxia: Asphyxia virtually certain. Marked increase in risk of perinatal mortality (125:1,000), so birth should be induced.
- Score – 0. Risk of fetal asphyxia: Certain asphyxia. Risk of perinatal mortality extremely high (600:1,000), so birth should be induced.

Fetal distress or complications

Fetal ultrasound is often used to evaluate fetal distress or complications:
- Placenta previa: Ultrasound is especially valuable in localizing the placenta, especially if it is implanted anteriorly or laterally, but if the placenta is in the lower posterior uterus, its position relative to the internal os is more difficult to identify. Because the placenta may move away from the os as the pregnancy develops, ultrasound allows for tracking and decision-making regarding method of delivery.
- Placenta abruptio: Ultrasound may help to exclude placenta previa as a cause of hemorrhage but otherwise is of little value in diagnosis.
- Multiple gestations: Serial ultrasounds are used to track multiple gestations. About 50% of cases in which twins are initially seen result in single births because of the death and reabsorption of one fetus. Chorionicity can be determined by week 9 or 10.
- Ruptured membranes /Oligohydramnios: Ultrasound can show decrease in amniotic fluid.

High Risks Factors Associated with Pregnancy

Classes I to IV cardiac disease

The New York Heart Association (NYHA) classifies heart disease by the functional capacity, and the maternal classification affects the fetus:
- I.   No cardiac insufficiency or activity limitations
- II. Slight limitation of activity with symptoms present with ordinary physical activity
- III. Marked limitation of activity; mild activity causes symptoms
- IV. Inability to carry out physical activities without severe symptoms

There is minimal danger to the fetus for mothers in class I or II but increased risk to both the mother and the fetus for classes III and IV. Most medications cross the placenta and the degree of safety during pregnancy is not always established, although most common drugs (heparin, digitalis glycosides, antiarrhythmics, thiazide and loop diuretics) are not teratogenic. For classes III and IV, delivery may be facilitated by low forceps or vacuum assistance, and cesarean may be done if the mother or fetus is in danger. Labor and delivery are particularly dangerous to the fetus because of inadequate oxygen and blood supply, so continuous fetal monitoring is essential.

Cardiopulmonary defects

With improved techniques of surgical repair of congenital heart defects, many women survive to childbearing age. Common maternal defects include tetralogy of Fallot, ventricular and atrial septal defects, patent ductus arteriosus, and coarctation of aorta. If surgical correction was successful, there is no added fetal risk, but if the condition was not completely repaired or involves cyanosis, pregnancy can put the fetus at risk because of inadequate oxygen supply (and 2% to 4% risk that the child will inherit the condition). Marfan syndrome poses severe risks to the mother with mortality rates of 25% to 50% because of possible rupture of the aorta, which also puts the fetus at risk. Additionally, because this is an autosomal dominant disorder, there is a 50% chance an infant will inherit. Mitral valve prolapse usually does not pose a risk to the fetus. Severe maternal cardiopulmonary disorders can result in death of the mother and/or fetus. However, the most common fetal complications are premature labor/birth and small for gestational age.

GDM

ADA (American Diabetes Association) Clinical Practice Recommendations for GDM (gestational diabetes) include the following screening and diagnostic procedures:
- Assessment of risk should be done at initial visit and further testing for those at high risk: obese, previous GDM or delivery of infant more than 9 pounds, glycosuria, PCOS, or family history of type 2 diabetes
- All women except those at very low risk should be tested at 14 to 28 weeks of gestation with one of two methods:
  - Plasma/serum glucose 1 hour after 50 g glucose load with more than 140 mg/dL (threshold), which will diagnose 80% of those with GDM. Those who exceed this threshold level should have a 100 g oral glucose tolerance test (OGTT) on another day

- 100 g OGTT in the morning after 8-hour fast with TWO of the following fasting glucose levels diagnostic of GDM: Fasting at least 95 mg/dL; 1 hour at least 180 mg/dL; 2 hours at least 155 mg/dL; 3 hour more than 140 mg/dL

Very low risk women are younger than 25 years with normal weight, no family or abnormal glucose history, no poor obstetrical outcomes, and no membership in a high-risk ethnic group.

Diabetes mellitus

About 2% of women have or develop diabetes mellitus during pregnancy. Factors that affect maternal health include change in dietary habit (such as inadequate intake because of nausea and diarrhea), changes in hormones that affect glucose metabolism, and increased renal blood flow that interferes with tubular reabsorption and results in increased glucosuria. All of these factors make control of diabetes more difficult. Mothers are at increased risk of diabetic ketoacidosis, pregnancy-induced hypertension (preeclampsia), and diabetic retinopathy. Polyhydramnios (more than 2,000 mL of amniotic fluid) occurs in about 10%, increasing the risk of abruptio placenta, premature labor, and postpartal uterine atony. The risk of spontaneous abortion increases markedly if glucose levels are poorly controlled. Urinary tract infections, including pyelonephritis, may occur. Patient education is important to help the mother maintain adequate control of glucose with fasting AM plasma glucose at 90 to 100 mg per 100 mL and less than 120 to 140 mg per 100 mL during the day. Diet recommendations include 35 kilocalories per kg of ideal body weight. Induction at week 38 or 39 is common.

HIV/AIDS

Women with HIV/AIDS taking antiretroviral drugs before conception should continue with the medications, although efavirenz is contraindicated because of teratogenic effects. If diagnosis occurs during the first trimester, then treatment should begin at that point or at the beginning of the second trimester. With treatment during pregnancy, the transmission rate from mother to fetus is about 2%. Usual treatment is 500 to 600 mg of zidovudine (ZDV) in 2 to 5 doses daily from week 14. Cesarean delivery poses less chance of HIV transmission for the neonate but increases the risk of maternal infection. Cesarean delivery is recommended if mother lacked adequate prenatal care, has a viral load unclear or more than 1,000 copies/mL at 36 weeks, or if the mother had not received antiretroviral drugs or had taken only ZDV or azidothymidine (AZT) during her pregnancy. IV ZDV is started 3 hours prior to cesarean delivery and used continuously through labor and delivery for vaginal delivery. HIV increases the risk of maternal and fetal infections.

Adolescent pregnancy

Adolescent mothers younger than 15 years are not at higher risk than those older than 20 if they have adequate prenatal care and follow guidelines and recommendations, but this is often not the case. Teenage mothers are more likely to smoke and to gain inadequate weight, increasing the likelihood of premature delivery, low-birth weight infants, iron deficiency anemia, and preeclampsia/eclampsia. Additionally, there is increased risk of cephalopelvic disproportion because the mother may not be fully matured physically. Adolescents and young adults (15 to 19) also have increased risk of sexually transmitted diseases (such as gonorrhea, herpes, chlamydia, and syphilis). Many also drink alcohol and take illicit drugs, increasing the incidence of fetal abnormalities. In many cases, the male partner is younger than 20 and has little education, lacks employments, and may not be able to provide emotional or financial support. Adolescent partners are usually of similar social and educational background as the mothers and have not completed development and are not prepared for fatherhood. The nurse should remain nonjudgmental and supportive, educating the adolescent and encouraging good prenatal care.

Adolescent responses to discovering pregnancy

Adolescent response to pregnancy varies with age:

- Ages ≤ 14 - Pregnancy may result from abuse, incest, or casual relationships, so the young mother rarely has a supportive partner. The girl is usually dependent of the parents, especially the mother, who often makes the decisions. The girl may be very self-conscious about body changes, lack self-esteem, and have little knowledge about physiology or pregnancy.
- Ages 15 to 17 - Pregnancy is more likely to result from an intimate relationship, but concern about peer or parental rejection is heightened. The mother is usually more knowledgeable about pregnancy and options (OTC pregnancy test, adoption, abortion) and may confirm pregnancy before confiding in others. The young mother and parents may differ in values related to terminating pregnancy/adoption.
- Ages 18 to 19 - This young mother is more likely to confirm pregnancy early and on her own with an OTC pregnancy kit, and has a better understanding of the consequences of pregnancy. Decisions about pregnancy depend on relationship with and support of partner and parents.

Pregnancy issues

Pregnancy issues differ between trimesters:

- First trimester - Confirmation of pregnancy is often delayed because of lack of awareness, denial, or fear. Physical changes (increased breast size) may cause embarrassment. Family (if told) may be angry, upset, unsupportive, and/or may pressure the mother to make a decision regarding abortion (pro or con).
- Second trimester - Changes in the body and quickening make it difficult for the teenager to ignore or deny pregnancy, but some try to hide pregnancy by wearing constrictive or baggy clothing and by dieting to retain prepregnancy weight. Family conflicts may arise as the family members learn about the pregnancy. The teenager may experience increased dependency and consider her own needs rather than the needs of the fetus.
- Third trimester - The teenager may be eager to get the pregnancy over with and is often fearful of or has nightmares about labor and delivery. Some may have trouble viewing the fetus as a separate being. Some, however, begin to prepare for childbirth by buying clothes or supplies for the baby.

Mature pregnancy

Many women have chosen to delay pregnancy, resulting in a marked increase in pregnant women older than 35. These mothers tend to be better educated and more financially secure than younger mothers. If the mother is in good health, pregnancy poses little increased risk; however, the risk of death associated with pregnancy does increase with age. Those older than 40 have about 5 times the risk as those 24 or younger. Additionally, those 35 and older are likely to have preexisting health problems, such as diabetes or hypertension, which increase risk. They are more likely to have a cesarean delivery, placenta previa, abruptio placentae, and spontaneous abortion. There may also be increased risk to the fetus. The incidence of Down syndrome increases with mothers older than 35 and more markedly older than 40, so these mothers are more likely to want genetic testing. Macrosomia and congenital malformations are also more common. Older mothers with unplanned pregnancies may be concerned about their age, long-term care of the child, retirement plans, and lifestyle changes.

Multiple births

Multiple births, such as twins, triplets, and quadruplets, are increasing in incidence because of fertility and increased maternal age. Multiple gestations are always considered high risk for both the fetuses and mother. Mothers may require bedrest during the last trimester, especially with at least 3 fetuses, and may require hospitalization for close monitoring during last month prior to delivery. Complications include:

- Fetal/Neonatal: Increased incidence of spontaneous abortion and neonatal death. Risk of cerebral palsy correlating with decreased gestational age. Increased risk of IUGR reduction. Increased disabilities related to premature status. Increased incidence of respiratory distress syndrome, necrotizing enterocolitis, IV hemorrhage, ROP, and PDA.
- Maternal: Severe hypertension/ preeclampsia (risk increases 2 to 3 times). Anemia (usually hemoglobin about 10 g/dL) from 20 weeks gestation. Iron deficiency anemia is common if serum ferritin concentration is low.

Preterm delivery (61%) with average gestational age in weeks of 28 (quadruplets), 33 (triplets), and 37 (twins). Increased PROM, incompetent cervix, uterine dysfunction, and malpresentation. Increased incidence of instrumental and cesarean births.

Pregnancy terms

Gravida – Any pregnancy (including present) regardless of duration/outcome.

Nulligravida – A woman who has never been pregnant.

Primigravida – A woman with her first pregnancy.

Multigravida – A woman in her at least second pregnancy.

Para – Delivery of live or stillborn fetus/neonate > 20 weeks gestation.

Nullipara – Woman who has not given birth > 20 weeks gestation

Primipara – A woman who has given birth, live or stillborn, one time > 20 weeks gestation.

Multipara – A woman who has given birth, live or stillborn, ? 2 times > 20 weeks gestation.

Grand multipara – A woman who has given birth, live or stillborn, ? 5 times > 20 weeks gestation.

Term – 38 to 48 weeks duration of pregnancy.

Gestation – Number of weeks since the first day of last menstrual period (LMP)

Abortion – Death of fetus < 20 weeks gestation.

Stillbirth – Death of fetus > 20 weeks gestation.

Grand multiparity

Grand multiparity is at least 5 deliveries of live or stillborn infants at least 20 weeks gestation, although some studies suggest risks increase after 4 deliveries. Great grand multiparity is usually considered at least 10 deliveries. Risks associated with multiparity include increased incidence of placenta previa, abruptio placentae, preeclampsia, and hemorrhage. Rates of cesarean deliveries are increased significantly. Grand multiparas often have poor prenatal care and tend to have increased rates of disease, such as diabetes mellitus and hypertension, but studies show that with proper prenatal care, those without health problems have risks comparable with those with lower parity. Younger multiparous women have fewer complications than older multiparous women, so some of the increased risks may be primarily age-related. Fetal complications include macrosomia, SGA, and malpresentation (breech).

Female infertility

Causes of female infertility are as follows:
- Nonpatent fallopian tubes - Fallopian tubes may be scarred by PID, endometrisis, or adhesions. Tests include hysterosalpingography and laparoscopy.
- Ovulation failure - Hormone levels may be inadequate to promote ovulation. Ovarian cysts may interfere with ovulation. Testing checks hormone levels of luteinizing hormone, progesterone, and prolactin and ultrasound (transvaginal) can be performed.
- Cervical obstruction or uterine abnormality - Excess production of mucous or narrowing of the cervical os may prevent sperm from entering the uterus. Thickening, abnormalities, or growths fibroids, cysts) of the uterus may prevent implantation. Tests include hysteroscopy, endometrial biopsy, postcoital test, and ultrasound (hysterosonogram).

Male fertility tests

Testing for male fertility includes the following:
- Urogenital history and examination - A history should review drug abuse, smoking, exercise, STDs, and sexual behaviors. The male is examined for physical abnormalities, such as varicocele, and the testes evaluated for size.
- Semen analysis - Usually two different semen samples, from different times, are examined. Two normal tests usually indicate the male is fertile. The sperm count is calculated and the sperm examined for size, shape, and motility.

- Hormone levels - Testosterone and other hormone levels may be evaluated, but abnormal hormone levels are associated with only about 3% of male infertility cases.
- Genetic testing - Testing may identify Klinefelter syndrome (male with an extra X chromosome) or Y microdeletion (cause of aspermia).

Assisted reproduction

The following are methods of assisted reproduction:
- Assisted reproduction therapy (ART) with egg and/or sperm donation - Donor eggs or sperm are combined with the partner's eggs or sperm before in intrauterine insemination.
- Gamete intrafallopian transfer (GIFT) - Sperm and ovum (gametes) are harvested/collected and inserted next to each other in the fallopian tube where normal fertilization takes place.
- Intracytoplasmic sperm injection (ICSI) - Individual harvested ovum is injected directly with individual sperm before intrauterine insemination. (May be part of ART.)
- Intrauterine insemination (IUI) - Sperm are inserted directly into the uterus through a catheter. This procedure may follow hormone treatments to stimulate ovulation.
- In vitro fertilization (IVF) - Fertilized ova are inserted into the uterus, often after the woman takes drugs to stimulate production of ova and harvesting. Ova and/or sperm may be donated.
- Zygote intrafallopian transfer (ZIFT) - Sperm and ova are combined and fertilization occurs outside the body, and then the zygotes are inserted into the fallopian tube where they travel to the uterus to implant.

Gonadotropin treatment

Gonadotropin treatment requires administration of natural or recombinant hormones: follicle-stimulating hormone (FSH) and luteinizing hormone (LH). Drugs include human chorionic gonadotropin (hCG), human menopausal gonadotropin (hMG), and recombinant human FSH (rFSH):
- Females who are not ovulating usually receive injections of hCG or hMG for 12 days to stimulate maturity of follicles and then 1 dose of hCG to trigger ovulation. About 60% become pregnant, but over half result in miscarriage. There is increased risk of multiple gestations, and ovarian enlargement or ovarian hyperstimulation syndrome may occur. Gonadotropins may also be used prior to harvesting of ova. Frequent ultrasounds and hormone levels are required to monitor the development of follicles.
- Males with low testosterone levels usually receive injections of hCG 3 times weekly for 4 to 6 months until testosterone levels increase. Then, men continue to receive injections of hCG or hMG 2 times weekly until sperm count is adequate. Gynecomastia may occur.

Fertility drugs

Bromocriptine reduces prolactin levels. Increased prolactin levels can interfere with ovulation in females and decrease testosterone levels and sperm production in males, resulting in impotence or erectile dysfunction. This drug is taken vaginally or orally 1 to 4 times daily, increasing the dose slowly to minimize adverse effects, which include headaches, dizziness, and GI disturbances. Cabergoline's actions are the same as bromocriptine, but cabergoline is only taken 1 to 2 times a week. Adverse effects are milder than bromocriptine, usually only headache. Clomiphene stimulates hormone production and ovulation in women whose estrogen levels and pituitary function are normal. Clomiphene is taken orally for 5 days during menstruation for 3 to 6 months with dosage adjusted according to results of clomiphene challenge test (FSH levels). Males may take clomiphene to increase sperm counts. Clomiphene is often used to stimulate production of multiple ova prior to harvesting. Gonadotropin-releasing hormone (GnRH) is administered prior to gonadotropin treatment to prevent pituitary from stimulating production of FSH and LH so production can be controlled.

Cytomegalovirus

Cytomegalovirus, a member of the herpes simplex virus group, can cause asymptomatic infection in women. More than 50% of women are seropositive and may have chronic infections that persist for years. Cytomegalovirus is the most common intrauterine viral infection. Cytomegalovirus can be transmitted placentally or cervically during delivery (infecting 2.5% or less of neonates) and can put the fetus at high risk, with death rates of 20% to 30% among infants born with symptoms. About 90% of survivors have neurological disorders, such as microcephaly, hydrocephalus, cerebral palsy, and/or intellectual disability. In less severe infections, symptoms (intellectual disability, hearing deficits, learning disabilities) may be delayed. Commonly, the neonate is small for gestational age (SGA). The brain and liver are commonly affected, but all organs can be infected. Multiple blood abnormalities can occur: anemia, hyperbilirubinemia, thrombocytopenia, and hepatosplenomegaly.

Herpes simplex virus

Most pregnant women infected with herpes simplex virus (HSV), usually type 2, are asymptomatic and unaware of infection. Most vertical transmissions occur when the neonate travels through a colonized birth canal. The risk of transmitting HSV during the birth process varies greatly, depending if the infection is a new infection (primary) or a secondary outbreak. The transmission rate from women with a primary HSV infection is approximately 50%, while the transmission rate is 1% to 2% if the infection is a recurrence of HSV. Signs of a neonatal infection with HSV include:
- Skin, eye, and mucous membrane blistering at 10 to 12 days of life.
- Disseminated disease may spread to multiple organs, leading to pneumonitis, hepatitis, and intravascular coagulation.
- Encephalitis may be the only presentation, with signs of lethargy, irritability, poor feeding, and seizures.

A mother with active herpes should deliver by cesarean section within 4 to 6 hours after membranes rupture. An infant that is inadvertently exposed to an active lesion should be treated with acyclovir.

Chlamydia

Chlamydia is the most common sexually transmitted disease in the United States and can be passed on at the time of birth if the infant is delivered vaginally and comes into contact with contaminated vaginal secretions. The organism responsible for this infection is *Chlamydia trachomatis.* Because the mother infected with this organism is usually asymptomatic, preventative care for the newborn is essential. The usual infection site for the newborn is the eye in the form of conjunctivitis. States now require all newborns be given a prophylactic dose of either erythromycin or tetracycline ointment in the eyes at birth to prevent this infection. While the antibiotic ointment stops the eye infection, a few infants exposed to the pathogen will develop pneumonitis and/or ear infection.

Syphilis

An infant can be exposed to the syphilis organism, *Treponema pallidum,* during gestation and become infected in utero starting with weeks 10 to 15 of gestation. Many infected fetuses abort spontaneously or are stillborn. The infant born infected with syphilis can be asymptomatic at birth or can have a full multisystem infection. An infant who is symptomatic may have nonviral hepatitis with jaundice, hepatosplenomegaly, pseudoparalysis, pneumonitis, bone marrow failure, myocarditis, meningitis, anemia, edema associated with nephritic syndrome, and a rash on the palms of the hands and soles of the feet. Other symptoms, such as interstitial keratitis and dental and facial abnormalities may occur as the child develops. Treatment involves an aggressive regimen of penicillin administration with frequent follow-up until blood tests are negative.

Neisseria gonorrhoeae

Neisseria gonorrhoeae infections are common and may result in recurrent infection, pelvic inflammatory disease (PID), chronic pain, and infertility. Women who become pregnant and have a history of gonorrhea with salpingitis are 7 to 10 times more likely to have an ectopic pregnancy. Signs of infection (dysuria and green, foul-smelling discharge from the urethra and the vagina) may occur 3 to 5 days after contact. However, many women are asymptomatic, especially on initial infection. About 15% of those infected develop PID, sometimes requiring hospitalization. Those with suspected or confirmed infections must be treated aggressively with a broad-spectrum antibiotic with follow-up cultures 3 to 5 days after completion of therapy. Women who have multiple sex partners or use illicit drugs are at increased risk of gonorrhea. Vaginal delivery increases risk to the neonate and can result in severe conjunctivitis, rupture of the globe, and blindness; however, routine prophylaxis (usually erythromycin ointment) to the neonate's eyes is effective treatment.

HPV

Human papilloma virus (HPV) comprises more than 100 viruses. About 40 are sexually transmitted and invade mucosal tissue, causing genital warts (condylomata). HPV infection causes changes in the mucosa, which can lead to cervical cancer. Most HPVs cause little or no overt symptoms, but infections are very common, especially in those 15 to 25 years. More than 99% of cervical cancers are caused by HPV and 70% are related to HPVs 16 and 18. The HPV vaccine, *Gardasil*, protects against HPVs 6, 11 (which cause genital warts), 16, and 18 (which cause cancer). Protection is only conveyed if the female has not yet been infected with these strains. The vaccine is currently recommended for females 26 years or younger. Active lesions are resistive to treatment during pregnancy. If lesions are extensive, cesarean delivery is recommended to avoid tearing and the need for suturing tissues with lesions, as well as to decrease transmission to the infant, who may develop laryngeal papillomata (although risk is small).

Complications of Pregnancy

Surgical termination of procedures

Termination of pregnancy may be done before the time of fetal viability (up to 24 weeks), but increasingly state regulations are limiting access to late-term abortions:
- Vacuum aspiration - 4 to 10 weeks. This may be done manually or by machine, with a cervical dilator used first and then a cannula passed into the uterus to suction the tissue.
- Suction curettage - 6 to 14 weeks. This is similar to vacuum aspiration, but a looped curettage is inserted into the uterus after the tissue is suctioned to remove any remnants.
- Dilation and extraction - 14 to 24 weeks. The cervix is dilated, and the fetus extracted by instrument, usually followed by suctioning to remove remnants. This procedure is common during the second trimester.
- Intact dilation and extraction - > 18 weeks. This "partial birth abortion" usually follows induced labor and removes the intact fetus via the cervix, but it requires prior feticide (intraamniotic or intrafetal digoxin or potassium chloride) to prevent live birth.
- Hysterectomy/ Hysterotomy - 12 to 24 weeks. This procedure is used only as a last resort (rare).

Medical termination of pregnancy

Medical procedures for termination of pregnancy can be used during the first trimester. Because medication-induced abortion always involves cramping and heavy bleeding, supervision should be available in case hemorrhage occurs. Mifepristone is administered orally on day 1 to block action of progesterone and change endometrium and then misoprostol vaginally or buccally on day 2 or 3 (or within 8 hours if bleeding is occurring) to cause contractions to help expel the embryo/fetus. Medical examination to ensure complete abortion is done after 7 days. Methotrexate injection is administered on day 1 to stop cell division and growth of the embryo followed by misoprostol vaginally on day 6 or 7 with examination on day 8 to ensure abortion is complete. In some cases, misoprostol or mifepristone may be used alone. If abortion is incomplete after medication-induced abortion, then suction and curettage may be necessary to remove retained tissue.

Spontaneous abortion

Vaginal bleeding during the first trimester of pregnancy may indicate spontaneous abortion, ectopic pregnancy, gestational trophoblastic disease, or infection. All women of childbearing age with an intact uterus presenting with abdominal pain or vaginal bleeding should be assessed for pregnancy. Abortion classifications:

- Threatened: Vaginal bleeding during first half of pregnancy without cervical dilatation.
- Inevitable: Vaginal bleeding with cervical dilatation.
- Incomplete: Incomplete loss of products of conception, usually between 6 to 14 weeks.
- Complete: Complete loss of products of conception, before 20 weeks.
- Missed: Death of fetus before 20 weeks without loss of products of conception within 4 weeks.
- Septic: Infection with abortion.

Diagnostic tests include:

- Pelvic examination.
- Laboratory tests: CBC, Rh factor, antibody screen, urinalysis, quantitative serum beta-hCG level.
- Ultrasound to rule out ectopic pregnancy.

Treatment includes:

- Suctioning of vaginal vault with Yankauer suction tip with pathologic examination of tissue.
- Evacuation of uterus for incomplete abortion.
- RhoGAM (50 to 150 mcg) for bleeding in unsensitized Rh-negative women.

Ectopic pregnancy

Ectopic pregnancy occurs when the fertilized ovum implants outside the uterus in an ovary, fallopian tube (the most common site), peritoneal cavity, or cervix. Diagnostic studies include vaginal exam, pregnancy test, transvaginal sonography (TVS) to rule out intrauterine pregnancy, and hCG titers (increase more slowly with ectopic pregnancy). Progesterone level more than 22 helps rule out ectopic pregnancy.

Early symptoms include:
- Indications of pregnancy: amenorrhea, breast tenderness, nausea, and vomiting.
- Positive Chadwick sign (blue discoloration of cervix).
- Positive Hegar sign (softening of isthmus).
- Bleeding may be the first indication as hormones fluctuate.
- Hormone hCG present in blood and urine.

Symptoms of rupture include:
- One-sided or generalized abdominal pain.
- Decreased hemoglobin and hematocrit.
- Hypotension with hemorrhage.
- Right shoulder pain because of irritation of the subdiaphragmatic phrenic nerve.

Treatment includes:
- Methotrexate IM or IV if unruptured and ≤ 3.5 cm in size to inhibit growth and allow body to expel.
- Laparoscopic linear salpingostomy or salpingectomy.

Preeclampsia and eclampsia

Pregnancy-induced hypertension (also called preeclampsia or toxemia) is a disorder that develops in approximately 5% of all pregnancies. The main features are elevated blood pressure and proteinuria that develop around 20 weeks of gestation. Initial treatment of preeclampsia is magnesium sulfate to prevent seizures in the mother. Eclampsia occurs with seizures. Severe cases may require the premature delivery of the infant to relieve the condition. The main detrimental effect on the fetus occurs because of longstanding hypertension that leads to uteroplacental vascular insufficiency, which impairs the transfer of nutrients and oxygen to the fetus, resulting in intrauterine fetal growth retardation (IUGR). Placental abruption also occurs more frequently. The IUGR is usually asymmetric (fetal head size is normal for gestational age). Infants who are born with IUGR and/or prematurity have increased morbidity and mortality. Treatment includes antihypertensive medications, such as thiazide, hydralazine, propranolol, labetalol, nifedipine and methyldopa, as well as anticonvulsants if seizures occur.

Hypertensive disorders of pregnancy

Hypertensive disorders of pregnancy comprise a continuum ranging from mild to severe:
- Hypertension: BP greater than 140/90 or 20 mm Hg increase in systolic or 10 mm diastolic. May be long-term or transient without signs of preeclampsia or eclampsia.
- Preeclampsia: Hypertension associated with proteinuria (300 mg per 24 hours) and edema (peripheral or generalized) or increase of at least 5 pounds of weight in 1 week after 20th week of gestation. Severe preeclampsia is BP ≥ 160/110. Symptoms include headache, abdominal pain, and visual disturbances.
- Eclampsia: Preeclampsia with seizures occurring at 20th week of gestation to 1 month after delivery.
- HELLP syndrome (hemolysis, elevated liver enzymes [AST and ALT], and low platelets [less than 100,000]). Usually accompanied by epigastric or right upper quadrant pain.

Treatments include:
- Chronic hypertension: Methyldopa beginning with 250 mg every 6 hours
- Preeclampsia, eclampsia, HELLP:
  - Delivery of fetus (may be delayed with mild preeclampsia if less than 37 weeks gestation)
  - Magnesium sulfate IV 4 to 6 g over 15 minutes initially and then 1 to 2 g per hour
- Antihypertensive drugs

FMH/transfusion

Fetomaternal hemorrhage (FMH) occurs in many pregnancies without any signs or symptoms. A small amount of fetal blood in the maternal circulation (1 to 2 mL) (fetomaternal transfusion) has no clinical significance. Massive FMH (blood loss greater than 30 mL) occurs in about 3 of every 1,000 pregnancies, and is a major cause of stillbirths. Neonates' blood volume ranges from 85 to 100 mL/kg, so 30 mL of blood loss represents 10% to 12% of the blood volume in a 3 kg neonate. Neonates may present with anemia. Risk factors for FMH include maternal trauma, placental abruption, placental tumors, third-trimester amniocentesis, fetal hydrops, and twinning. One test used to diagnose the presence of FMH is the Kleihauer-Betke (KB) test, in which a sample of the mother's blood is examined for the presence of fetal hemoglobin. The KB test estimates the amount of hemorrhage that has taken place.

Abruptio placentae

With abruptio placentae, the placenta prematurely detaches, partially or completely, from the uterus. Abruptio placenta is related to maternal hypertension and incidence increases with cocaine abuse. Partial detachment interferes with the functioning of the placenta, causing intrauterine growth retardation. Severe bleeding occurs with total detachment. Diagnosis includes ultrasound, CBC and type and cross match, and coagulation studies (50% have coagulopathy).

Symptoms include:
- Vaginal bleeding.
- Tender uterus with increased resting tone.
- Uterine contractions (hypertonic or hyperactive.
- Nausea and vomiting (in some patients).
- Dizziness.
- Complications include fetal distress, hypotension, and DIC, as well as fetal and/or maternal death.
- Fetal death common with at least 50% separation.
- Irreversible brain damage may occur with fetal hypoxia, and neurological deficits occur in about 14% of survivors.

Treatment includes:
- Gynecological consultation.
- Crystalloids to increase blood volume.
- Fresh frozen plasma for coagulopathy.
- Partial: Bedrest and monitoring.
- Complete: Immediate vaginal or cesarean delivery.

Placenta previa

Placenta previa occurs when the placenta implants over or near the internal cervical os. Implantation may be complete (covering the entire opening), partial, or marginal (to the edge of the cervical opening). Women with placenta previa have increased incidences of hemorrhage in the third trimester. Symptoms include painless bleeding after 20th week of gestation. Diagnosis is by ultrasound. Vaginal examination with digit or speculum should be avoided. The condition may correct itself as the uterus expands, but bed rest may be needed. Emergency cesarean delivery is done for uncontrolled bleeding. In infants, placenta previa is associated with poor growth, anemia, and increased risk of congenital anomalies in their central nervous systems, heart, respiratory, and gastrointestinal tracts. Placenta previa may also cause premature birth with associated neonatal complications of prematurity.

DIC

Disseminated intravascular coagulation (DIC) (consumption coagulopathy) is a secondary disorder of pregnancy. DIC may be triggered by abruptio placentae, uterine rupture, embolism of amniotic fluid, eclampsia, postpartum hemorrhage, shock (hypovolemic), severe infection with sepsis, or saline/missed abortion. DIC triggers both coagulation and hemorrhage through a complex series of events that includes trauma that causes tissue factor (transmembrane glycoprotein) to enter the circulation and bind with coagulation factors, triggering the coagulation cascade. This stimulates thrombin to convert fibrinogen to fibrin, causing aggregation and destruction of platelets and forming clots that can be disseminated throughout the intravascular system. These clots increase in size as platelets adhere to the clots, causing blockage of both the microvascular systems and larger vessels, and this can result in ischemia and necrosis. Clot formation triggers fibrinolysis and plasmin to breakdown fibrin and fibrinogen, causing destruction of clotting factors, resulting in hemorrhage. Both processes, clotting and hemorrhage, continue at the same time, placing the patient at high risk for death, even with treatment.

<u>Symptoms and treatment</u>
The onset of symptoms of DIC may be very rapid or a slower chronic progression from a disease. Those who develop the chronic manifestation of the disease usually have fewer acute symptoms and may slowly develop ecchymosis or bleeding wounds. Symptoms include:
- Bleeding from surgical or venous puncture sites.
- Evidence of GI bleeding with distention, bloody diarrhea.
- Hypotension and acute symptoms of shock.
- Petechiae and purpura with extensive bleeding into the tissues.
- Laboratory abnormalities:
  - Prolonged prothrombin and partial prothrombin times.
  - Decreased platelet counts and fragmented RBCs.
  - Decreased fibrinogen.

Treatment includes:
- Identifying and treating underlying cause.
- Replacement blood products, such as platelets and fresh frozen plasma.
- Anticoagulation therapy (heparin) to increase clotting time.
- Cryoprecipitate to increase fibrinogen levels.
- Coagulation inhibitors and coagulation factors.

Hyperemesis gravidarum

About 60% to 80% of pregnant woman suffer from nausea and vomiting (NV), especially during the first trimester, but only about 2% suffer severe (sometimes intractable) nausea and vomiting, known as hyperemesis gravidarum (HG). Nausea and vomiting may be associated with numerous disorders, including cholelithiasis, pancreatitis, hepatitis, and ectopic pregnancy, especially if accompanied by abdominal pain. Diagnosis includes physical examination to rule out other disorders, CBC with serum electrolytes, BUN, creatinine, and urinalysis.

Symptoms include:
- Severe (sometimes intractable) NV
- Weight loss
- Dehydration
- Hypokalemia
- Ketonemia
- Ketonuria (indication of inadequate nutrition)

Treatment includes:
- IV fluids with 5% glucose in normal saline or lactated Ringer's
- Oral fluids after nausea and vomiting controlled.
- Antiemetic drugs
  - Acute treatment for NV and HG: promethazine, prochlorperazine, or chlorpromazine
  - Maintenance for NV: Doxylamine with pyridoxine, diphenhydramine, or cisapride
  - Maintenance for HG: Metoclopramide, trimethobenzamide, or ondansetron

Hydatidiform mole

Hydatidiform mole (molar pregnancy) results from gestational trophoblastic disease, the pathologic proliferation of trophoblastic cells (specialized cells in the blastocyst around an embryo that develop into the placenta). Hydatidiform mole results in loss of pregnancy, often through spontaneous abortion. There are two types of molar pregnancy:
- **Complete:**
  - An anuclear ("empty") ovum usually is fertilized with a 23X haploid sperm and duplicates before cell division, resulting in a 46XX mole of completely paternal origin.
  - Avascular hydropic vesicles form from chorionic villi, all of which are edematous.
  - No embryonic or fetal tissue is present.
  - Choriocarcinoma may develop (15% to 30%).
- **Partial:**
  - A normal ovum is fertilized by 2 sperm or by a sperm that still contains 46 chromosomes, resulting in a mole with 69 chromosomes. In some cases, the ovum still contains 46 chromosomes and is fertilized by a normal sperm.
  - Vascular hydropic vesicles form in areas of the placenta rather than throughout.
  - The abnormal fetus may survive to 8 or 9 weeks.
  - Choriocarcinoma rare (< 5%).

The following are symptoms of hydatidiform mole:
- Uterine size - Uterus is enlarged in 50% of cases of complete mole but may be too small for gestation in other cases. Enlargement is caused by proliferating trophoblastic tissue and clotted blood. On ultrasound, the mole has a "snowstorm" appearance.
- Bleeding - Vaginal bleeding occurs in almost all molar pregnancies, usually by 4 weeks but may occur in the second trimester. Bleeding may be brownish "prune juice" in appearance or bright red.
- Tissue passage - Hydropic vesicles may be passed vaginally, especially with complete mole.
- Fetal heart sounds - Absence of fetal heart sounds is a classic indication of molar pregnancy, although in some cases a partial mole may have a fetal heart sound.
- Pregnancy tests - Positive.
- hCG titers - High with complete mole and moderately high to high with partial.

Rh incompatibility

Rh incompatibility occurs if the mother is Rh- and the father is Rh+, putting their infant is at risk for hemolytic disease of the newborn (HDN) or Rh disease (erythroblastosis fetalis). Sensitization can occur during abortion, abruptio placenta, amniocentesis, cesarean section, chorionic villus sampling, cordocentesis, delivery, ectopic pregnancy, and toxemia. To prevent erythroblastosis fetalis, women who are Rh- with an Rh+ mate receive the serum *RhoGAM*, containing anti-Rh+ antibodies. The purpose of the antibodies is to agglutinate any fetal red blood cells that pass over into the mother's circulatory system and thus prevent the mother from forming antibodies against them that will attack the infant and sensitize her for future pregnancies.
- Mother receives 300 mcg of *RhoGAM* (Rh immunoglobulin [RhIg]) IM at 26 to 28 weeks of pregnancy and again within 72 hours after her delivery
- Miscarriage, ectopic, abortion: At 12 weeks or fewer, the mother receives 50 mcg of *MICRhoGAM*. At 13 weeks or fewer, the mother receives *RhoGAM* as for pregnancy

ABO incompatibility is similar but usually less severe, although some infants require phototherapy for jaundice and/or exchange transfusion.

Intrapartal Period

Normal Labor

Latent and active phases

The stages of labor present somewhat differently from one woman to another and in multipara and nullipara:
- First stage: This stage signals onset of labor with regular contractions and proceeds until the cervix is fully dilated. There are 3 phases:
- Latent: This early phase may persist for 8.5 hours for nullipara and 5.3 hours for the multipara. The cervix begins to dilate (3 cm or less) and contractions may occur every 3 to 30 minutes, lasting 20 to 40 seconds. The intensity of the contractions is usually mild to moderate (25 to 40 mm Hg per intrauterine pressure catheter [IUPC]). The mother is usually able to cope with discomfort and may feel some anxiety.
- Active: This phase may persist for 4.5 hours in the nullipara but 2.5 hours in the multipara. The cervix dilates to 4 to 7 cm (1.2 cm/hour for nullipara and 1.5 cm/hour for multipara) with contractions increasing in frequency every 1 to 5 minutes with duration of 40 to 60 seconds. The intensity is moderate to strong (50 to 70 mm Hg per IUPC) and anxiety and pain increase.

Transition phase

After the latent and active phases, the last phase of the first stage of labor is transition. This phase may persist for 3.6 hours for the nullipara and 1 hour or less for the multipara, although this duration may increase an hour with epidural anesthesia. The cervix becomes fully dilated to 8 to 10 cm with frequent contractions every 1.5 to 2 minutes lasting 60 to 90 seconds. The intensity is strong by palpation and 70 to 90 mm Hg per IUPC. During this stage, the mother may experience much anxiety and pain and the feeling that bearing down or contractions will tear her apart. Cervical dilation slows between 8 to 10 cm and fetal descent increases (1 cm/hour for nullipara and 2 cm/hour for multipara). Mothers frequently request pain medication and may hyperventilate, have difficulty following directions, cry or moan, become very restless, hiccup, belch or vomit, and complain of rectal pressure.

Second stage of labor

The second stage of labor begins when the cervix is fully dilated and ends with delivery. This stage usually lasts for about 2 hours for the nullipara but only 15 minutes for the multipara. Frequent contractions continue every 1.5 to 2 minutes and last 60 to 90 seconds (as in transition phases of stage 1), and intensity is very strong by palpation and 70 to 100 mm Hg by IUPC. As the fetal head descends, it applies pressure to the sacral and obturator nerves, causing an intense urge to bear down. The perineum begins to bulge and flatten out and bloody show increases. The mother often feels severe pain and burning in the perineal area. The fetal head crowns as delivery is imminent. The perineum thins as the fetal head distends the vulva and the anus, sometimes causing stool to be expelled. The head is born and then the shoulders and body in a spontaneous (non-breech) birth.

Third and fourth stages of labor

The third stage of labor commences after the delivery of the infant and ends after the placenta is delivered. After delivery, strong uterine contractions decrease surface area of placental attachment, causing separation, which is accompanied by bleeding and formation of a hematoma between the decidua and the placental tissue. Finally, the placental membrane peels off of the uterine wall. Signs of placental separation usually occur between 5 and 30 minutes after birth:
- Globular-shaped uterus
- Fundus rises in the abdomen
- Increased gush or trickling of blood
- Umbilical cord protrudes further from the vagina

A placenta is considered retained if it has not separated in more than 30 minutes after delivery. The fourth stage is the time period extending from 1 to 4 hours after birth during which the mother's body goes through physiologic readjustment. Blood is redistributed and this, coupled with 250 to 400 mL of blood loss, contributes to moderate hypotension and tachycardia. The uterus stays contracted, and the fundus is usually midline between the symphysis pubis and umbilicus.

Assessing progress of labor and vital signs

During the first stage of labor, the following assessments are made:
- Initial admission exam:
  - Contractions: Frequency and duration and changes are noted since onset.
  - Cervical exam: Dilatation may vary from 1 to 10 cm with multipara averaging dilatation of 1.2 cm/h and multipara 1.5 cm/h. Effacement varies from 0 to 100%. Fetal descent may range from +4 to -4.
- Latent phase:
  - Check baseline VS and then monitor every hour if stable (90 to 140/60 to 90) or every 15 minutes if unstable or elevating > 30 mm Hg systolic/> 15 mm Hg diastolic over baseline.
  - Monitor temperature every 4 hours. If > 37.6°C or membranes rupture, monitor every 2 hours.
  - Monitor uterine contractions every 30 minutes (usually occur every 5 to 10 minutes with duration of 15 to 40 seconds, mild intensity.).
  - Monitor FHR every 60 minutes for low-risk mothers and every 30 minutes for high-risk mothers if FHR remains within normal range (110 to 160). If FHR unstable, use continuous monitoring.
- Active phase:
  - Check VS every hour if stable or every 15 minutes if unstable.
  - Monitor temperature every 4 hours. If > 37.6°C or membranes rupture, monitor every 2 hours.
  - Monitor uterine contractions every 15 to 30 minutes (usually occur every 2 to 3 minutes with duration of 60 seconds, moderate intensity).

- o Monitor FHR every 30 minutes for low-risk mothers and every 15 minutes for high-risk mothers if FHR within normal range. Institute interventions as necessary if FHR is unstable.
  - o Monitor mother's comfort level and coping mechanisms.
  - o Monitor response to analgesia/anesthesia.
- Transition phase:
  - o Check VS every 30 minutes.
  - o Monitor uterine contractions every 15 minutes (usually occur every 2 minutes with duration of 60 to 75 seconds, strong intensity).
  - o Monitor bladder distention. Use straight catheter if unable to urinate.
  - o Continue monitoring comfort level, coping mechanisms, and response to analgesia/anesthesia.

During the second stage the following assessments are made:
- Check VS every 5 to 15 minutes.
- Monitor uterine contractions continuously
- Monitor FHR every 15 minutes for low-risk mothers and every 5 minutes for high-risk mothers. If unstable, monitor continuously.
- Monitor fetal descent.
- Monitor mother's comfort level and coping mechanisms.
- Monitor response to analgesia/anesthesia.
- Monitor bladder distention. Use straight catheter if unable to urinate.

During the third stage of labor the following assessments are made:
- Check VS every 5 minutes.
- Continue to monitor all aspects of labor and delivery.
- Monitor uterine contractions every few minutes or as indicated until the placenta is delivered.
- Monitor response to analgesia/anesthesia (epidural, spinal).
- Provide support during pudendal local anesthesia and episiotomy if indicated.
- Monitor bladder distention. Use straight catheter if unable to urinate.

Birth plan

Having a birth plan prepared can alleviate much of the stress associated with labor because it allows the mother and her partner to make decisions in advance about what she wants during labor and delivery. Elements that should be included in a birth plan are:
- Labor - Specific preferences regarding ambulation during the labor process and IVs or oral fluids. May also indicate how frequently the mother wants vaginal exams.
- Fetal monitoring - Desire for continuous fetal monitoring or intermittent.
- Induction - Conditions under which induction procedures or other procedures to speed up labor, such as artificial rupturing of the membranes, are acceptable.
- Anesthesia/Comfort measures - Preferences for natural childbirth, opiates only, epidural, or spinal anesthesia. May include any birth preparation methods the mother plans to use, such as Lamaze.
- Surgical interventions - Specific conditions for cesarean delivery or episiotomy.
- Delivery - Instructions regarding positioning, pushing, mirror, support (partner, friend, husband), and immediate care of newborn.

- Postpartal period - Includes preferences regarding cutting cord, rooming in, nursery care, private or shared room, breastfeeding, supplementary feeding, and disposing/donating cord blood.

Progressive relaxation

Progressive relaxation is one method to help the mother relax her muscles and relieve tension so that uterine contractions are more effective. Progressive relaxation involves first tightening muscles and holding the tension for a few seconds and then relaxing them, concentrating on the difference in feeling between the tense and relaxed muscle states and imagining the tension flowing out of the muscles. Relaxation is usually done bilaterally, starting with the feet and moving upward through the muscles of the lower legs, the hands, the lower arms, the upper arms, and finally the abdomen and chest, the neck, and the face.

Vocalization

Vocalization is a technique that encourages the woman to make sounds during contractions in order to relieve tension and relax muscles. The woman is coached to drop her jaw and try to make low-pitched (masculine sounding) moans as this method opens the glottis and makes breathing easier. High-pitched moaning should be avoided as it may increase tension.

Touch relaxation

Touch relaxation requires a coach and is generally practiced prior to onset of labor. The mother learns to relax her muscles in response to touch—first her partner's and later doctors' and nurses'. In this technique, the mother tightens a small area of muscles, and her coach gently strokes the area, "pulling" the tension away as the mother immediately relaxes the muscles at the first touch. Strokes are generally in a downward direction. Touch relaxation follows a specific sequence, and a printed guide may be helpful for the woman and her coach. The sequence of contracting and relaxing begins with the scalp and eyebrows, the rest of the face and jaw, the shoulder blades, abdomen, thighs, legs, and arms. After the initial sequence, the mother lies on her side, tightening the back of the neck, which the coach then strokes and massages. Then, she curls into fetal position and tightens the upper back, lower back, and buttocks.

Dissociation relaxation

Dissociation relaxation is a method that teaches the mother to tighten just one set of voluntary muscles and relax the rest (neuromuscular dissociation) to prepare the mother to relax all voluntary muscles during uterine contractions. This technique uses discomfort to help the mother dissociate from the pain. For example, the partner may grasp the upper arms and rotate the skin outward to create a burning sensation in the muscles or pinch an area of the inner thigh (being careful not to injure the woman or cause real pain). Then, the woman relaxes other muscles in a sequence of contracting, holding, and relaxing. The partner touches the relaxed muscles to check relaxation. The usual sequence is right arm, left arm, right leg, left leg, both arms, both legs, right arm and leg, and finally left arm and leg.

Visualization

There are a number of methods used for visualization. Some include audiotapes with guided imagery, such as self-hypnosis tapes, but the pregnant woman can be taught basic techniques that include:

- Lie on back or left side (preferred) in a quiet place (if possible), eliminating unnecessary distractions
- Concentrate on breathing while taking long slow breaths
- Close the eyes to shut out distractions and create an image in the mind of the place or situation desired
- Concentrate on that image, engaging as many senses as possible, and imaging details.
- If the mind wanders, breathe deeply and bring consciousness back to the image, or concentrate on breathing for a few moments and then return to the imagery
- End with positive imagery

Sometimes, women in labor are resistive at first or have a hard time maintaining focus, so guiding them through visualization for the first few times can be helpful.

Labor comfort measures

Comfort measures during labor include the following:

- Positioning - Mothers are often encouraged to ambulate during the first stage of labor, but if the FHR is not reassuring or if the membranes are ruptured, the mother may be confined to bed or chair. In that case, she should be helped to turn at least every hour or to sit in a warm shower or rocking chair to increase relaxation and relieve discomfort. If in bed, the body, arms, and legs should be supported comfortably with pillows or bolsters with joints slightly flexed. If the mother prefers the supine position, the head of the bed should be elevated to at least 30 degrees and support placed under the lower back to relieve uterine pressure on the vena cava.
- Hydrotherapy - Shower, warm bath, and whirlpool all help to relax the mother and reduce discomfort. Tub bath and whirlpool, however, should be avoided if the membranes have ruptured.
- Perineal care - Increased vaginal discharge can cause odor and discomfort, so the perineal pad should be changed at least every hour and the perineum gently washed with warm water and soap to remove secretions.
- Hydration - Diaphoresis, the effort expended during labor, and breathing patterns often cause the mother to feel thirsty and complain of dry mouth. If allowed, clear fluids should be offered; otherwise, ice chips or hard candy may be used.
- Skin care (Diaphoresis)- Increased perspiration and amniotic leakage often leave the woman's bedclothes damp and cold, so frequent gown and linen changes should be done. Underpads can be placed under the buttocks and changed frequently as they are more easily changed than the bottom sheet. A cool damp cloth on the forehead may be soothing.
- Bladder emptying - The mother may be unable to completely empty the bladder because of fetal pressure or discomfort, but a distended bladder will add to her discomfort during contractions. The mother should be encouraged to try urinating every 1 to 2 hours, preferably on the toilet, as it may be more difficult to empty the

bladder on a bedpan. If the mother is unable to urinate or completely empty her bladder and her bladder remains distended, a straight catheterization may be necessary, although repeated catheterizations increase the risk of infection.

- Birthing balls - Sitting with the legs spread apart on a birthing ball and slowly rocking back and forth helps to increase pelvic diameter and facilitate fetal descent. The mother should not be left unattended while on the ball as she may lose balance or fall.

Opioids and sedatives

Opioids and sedatives are usually given only in the early stages of labor, sometimes with patient-controlled analgesia (PCA), because they readily cross the placental barrier and can cause central nervous system depression in the fetus. This depression can persist after delivery, especially in premature infants, affecting Apgar scores. Some drugs, such as morphine and benzodiazepines, are avoided because of excessive fetal depression.

Drugs used include:
- Meperidine (1 to 25 mg IV or 25 to 50 mg IM to maximum 100 mg) is the most common. IV onset is 1 to 20 minutes and IM 1 to 3 hours, and its use is limited to more than 4 hours before delivery.
- Fentanyl (25 to 100 mcg/h IV) has shorter onset (3 to 10 minutes) with 1-hour duration and causes less fetal depression.
- Butorphanol 1 to 2 mg or nalbuphine 10 to 20 mg IV or IM causes little respiratory effect and provides adequate relief of pain but may result in excessive sedation if given repeatedly.
- Promethazine (25 to 50 mg IM) and hydroxyzine may be used in combination with meperidine or alone to provide relief of anxiety and reduce dose of opioid.

Pudendal nerve block

Visceral pain occurs in the first stage of labor from contractions and cervical dilation with afferent impulses entering the spinal cord at T10 to T11. However, during the second stage of labor, the stretching of the vagina and perineum caused by descent of the fetus causes somatic pain with impulses carried by the pudendal nerves to the spinal cord at S2 to S4. Pudendal nerve block is used during the second stage (sometimes along with perineal infiltration) to reduce somatic pain when neuraxial blocks are contraindicated and for episiotomy and relaxation of the pelvic floor for forceps delivery. With the patient in lithotomy position, a transvaginal or transperineal approach is used to block the nerve. For the transvaginal approach (the most common), a special guide, Kobak needle or Iowa trumpet, is used to prevent inadvertent injection into the fetal head. Anesthetic agents include 10 mL of 1% lidocaine or 2% chloroprocaine. The transperineal approach may be used if the head is engaged.

Lumbar epidural

The most common form of regional anesthesia/analgesia for labor and delivery is the lumbar epidural. Dilute mixtures of local anesthetic and opioids are combined. The catheter is usually placed early so that it is available when pain relief is needed. At one time, epidurals were delayed until labor was well established, but current trends are to administer earlier if the fetus is in no distress, contractions are 3 to 4 minutes and persisting at least 60 seconds, and the fetal head is engaged with 3 to 4 cm of cervical dilation. The catheter is usually placed with the mother in sitting position to ensure sacral spread. Placement is usually at L3 to L4 or L4 to L5. If inadvertent spinal placement occurs, spinal anesthesia/analgesia may be given or the catheter removed and replaced at a higher level. Most commonly, bupivacaine or ropivacaine (0.0625% to 0.125%) is given in combination with fentanyl (2 to 3 mcg/mL) or sufentanil (0.3 to 0.5 mcg/mL). If dilute anesthetic agents are used, the mother may be able to ambulate while receiving the epidural.

Epidural analgesia with opioids

Epidural analgesia with just opioids is also sometimes used during the first stage of labor. Commonly used agents include morphine (5 mg), meperidine (50 to 100 mg), fentanyl (50 to 150 mcg), and sufentanil (10 to 20 mcg). The duration of analgesia is longer with administration of epidural opioids than with intrathecal, but many of the same problems occur. Low doses of morphine may not provide adequate pain relief and higher doses may cause respiratory depression. Morphine has a slow onset (30 minutes to 1 hour) but provides analgesia for 12 to 24 hours. Meperidine provides good relief but is short-acting (1 to 3 hours). Fentanyl and sufentanil both have rapid onset but are also short acting (1 to 2 hours). Commonly, morphine is combined with fentanyl or sufentanil for fast onset with long duration. The fetus must be monitored carefully if repeated epidural doses of opioids are administered as they can cause fetal depression.

Intrathecal analgesia with opioids

Intrathecal (spinal) analgesia (into the subarachnoid space) with just opioids is sometimes used during the first stage of labor. Commonly used agents include morphine (0.25 to 0.5 mg), meperidine (10 to 15 mg), fentanyl (12.5 to 15 mcg), and sufentanil (92 to 10 mcg). Meperidine is the only agent that has local anesthetic characteristics. Higher doses are needed if spinal opioids are used alone, administered as a single dose or intermittently per catheter, and this can result in higher risk of complications, maternal respiratory depression, and fetal depression. However, if given alone, opioids (except for meperidine) do not provide motor blockade or maternal hypotension, so the mother is able to push. However, the analgesic effect may not be adequate, and adverse effects (pruritus, nausea, and vomiting) related to the agent may occur. Morphine alone has a slow onset (45 to 60 minutes), although it provides 4 to 6 hours of analgesia with spinal administration, but low doses may not provide adequate relief and high doses increase adverse effects. Morphine is frequently combined with fentanyl for more rapid onset. Commonly, opioids are combined with local anesthetics.

FHR

Fetal heart rate (FHR) monitoring is usually done by electronic fetal monitoring (EFM), as it provides a continuous tracing. FHR can be assessed by auscultation or ultrasound with an abdominal transducer, but tracings can be poor with an active fetus, with maternal movement, and with hydramnios. Intermittent monitoring is usually every 15 minutes in the first stage of labor and every 5 minutes in the second. Internal monitoring requires cervical dilation of at least 2 cm so that an electrode can be applied to the fetal presenting part (head or buttocks). Internal scalp electrodes should not be used if the mother has a communicable disease, such as HIV, or with preterm infants. Telemetry with ultrasound or

- 49 -

fetal ECG transducers and external uterine pressure transducers can also be used to monitor FHR. This type of battery-operated monitoring can be used while the mother ambulates, as it is less invasive. FHR patterns are evaluated based on a baseline rate (rate for 10 minutes between contractions), usually 110 to 160 bpm. Bradycardia is a rate less than 120 bmp and tachycardia greater than 160 bpm.

Fetal scalp sampling and stimulation

Fetal scalp sampling involves making a small cut in the fetal scalp and collecting a blood sample to monitor blood gas and pH. Fetal scalp sampling is used to determine if the fetus is receiving enough oxygen during labor, to measure fetal platelets, and to rule out acidosis. This technique has several limiting factors, such as inadequate cervical dilation, fetal head too high, membranes still intact, or sampling errors due to hematoma of the fetus's scalp. The results of the sampling are normal if the pH is greater than 7.25, pre-pathological if between 7.2 to 7.25, and pathological if less than 7.2. The test must be repeated every 20 to 30 minutes because the results are time-limited. Fetal scalp stimulation is done during the vaginal examination by gently massaging the scalp for 15 seconds. The results of scalp stimulation should be an increase in the fetal heart rate of 10 to 15 beats over baseline for 10 to 15 seconds. Failure of the heartbeat to accelerate is an indication of acidosis.

Tachycardia and bradycardia

Fetal heart rate usually varies with accelerations and decelerations. Fetal reactivity (accelerated fetal heart rate with fetal activity) begins at about 32 weeks gestation. Heart rate often increases for periods of 20 to 40 minutes. Causes for accelerated or decelerated fetal heart rate include:
- Tachycardia: greater than 160 for at least 10 minutes, severe greater than 180. Transient tachycardia occurs for less than 10 minutes and is usually not significant. Tachycardia may result from early fetal hypoxia, prematurity, medications (such as terbutaline), fetal infection, maternal fever, and anxiety.
- Bradycardia: less than 120 for at least 10 minutes, severe less than 80. Bradycardia at 100 to 119 is usually not significant, but bradycardia may indicate heart block or placentae abruptio. Uterine contractions slow fetal heart rate because of compression of the head affecting cerebral blood flow, compression of the myometrial vessels of the uterus, and/or occlusion of the umbilical cord causing fetal hypertension or hypoxemia. Medications (such as narcotics and oxytocin) and epidural anesthesia may cause decreased heart rate as well.

FHR and accelerations

Fetal heart rate variability shows sensitivity to oxygenation and acid-base status. Good variability indicates adequate oxygenation of the fetus's CNS. Decreased variability corresponds to fetal hypoxia and acidemia. Fetal heart rate variability is fluctuations in the fetal heart rate of 2 cycles or more, graded according to the range of amplitude.
- Absent: Range not detectable
- Minimal: 5 bpm or less
- Moderate: 6 to 25 bpm
- Marked: greater than 25 bpm

Short-term variability is a variation in amplitude of 3 to 8 bpm on a beat-to-beat basis. Long-term variability is an irregular pattern of variability of 3 to 5 cycles/min with amplitude of 5 to 15 bpm. FHR accelerations are transient increases in fetal heart rate. Nonperiodic accelerations relate to fetal movement. Periodic accelerations accompany contractions and/or compression of the umbilical cord and may indicate low amniotic fluid or dangerous cord compression.

FHR decelerations

Decelerations are transient decreases in FHR. They are categorized according to contraction cycle and waveform:
- Early: Caused by head compression as it descends the birth canal. Waveform is uniform with onset just before or at onset of contraction and lowest level at midpoint of contraction, inversely mirroring contraction. Range is usually 120 to 160 bpm. Deceleration may occur once or may repeat.
- Late: Caused by compression of vessels and uteroplacental insufficiency. Waveform is uniform with shape reflecting contraction. Onset is late in the contraction and lowest point is after midpoint of contraction. Range is 120 to 130 bpm. Deceleration may be occasional, consistent, or repetitive.
- Variable: Caused by umbilical cord compression. Waveform is variable with sharp drops and increases. Onset may be abrupt with fetal insult and not related to contraction. The lowest point is around the midpoint. The range is usually outside normal. Deceleration may be variable and occur once or repetitively. If they occur repetitively, this may indicate fetal distress.

Complications of Labor

Shoulder dystocia

Shoulder dystocia occurs when the head has been delivered but the infant's shoulder is wedged behind the mother's symphysis pubis. Shoulder dystocia is sometimes associated with macrosomia, post term pregnancies, gestational diabetes, protracted labor, or assisted vaginal delivery. Special precautions are indicated during delivery. If meconium is noted, then the infant's nose and mouth should be suctioned before the infant's shoulders are delivered. Maneuvers used to facilitate delivery include:
- Get help immediately
- Consider episiotomy
- Do McRoberts maneuver: The thighs are lifted and hyperflexed to elevate the pubic bone
- Apply suprapubic pressure externally over the wedged shoulder while traction is continued
- Manually rotate the infant's head and upper body while continuing suprapubic pressure
- Pull the posterior arm out of the birth canal, flex the elbow, and deliver the forearm over the chest wall

Cephalopelvic/fetopelvic disproportion

Cephalopelvic/fetopelvic disproportion is usually diagnosed when labor does not progress, although in rare cases it may be diagnosed prior to labor. It may relate to pelvic diameters that are too small (most common with android and platypelloid pelvic types) or contractures of the pelvic inlet (less than 10 cm anteroposterior diameter or less than 12 cm transverse diameter), contracted midpelvis, or contracted outlet (less than 8 cm interischial tuberous diameter). Rarely is this disproportion caused by excessive fetal size as most fetuses are within normal size and weight limits. Usually labor is extended, and premature rupture of the membranes occurs, increasing danger of cord prolapse. The fetal head is often markedly molded and continued pressure can cause neurological injury or even death of the fetus if the labor continues and the fetus cannot be delivered. However, when labor fails to progress, the mother is usually given a cesarean section (2 hours or less of labor onset) to prevent further injury to the fetus.

Multiple gestations

In vitro fertilization and ovulation-inducing drugs have increased the incidence of high-order multiple gestations over the past 30 years. The trend of delayed childbearing has led to an increase in twin/multiple gestations. Infants born from multiple gestations are more likely to be born prematurely and with low birth weights. The incidence of premature birth and low birth weight is proportional to the number of fetuses. There may be growth restriction/growth discordance, oligohydramnios, and restriction of movement of 1 or more fetuses. Approximately 50% of twins and 90% of triplets are born premature, compared with 10% of singletons. With this increase in prematurity and proportion of infants born with low birth weight, there are increased morbidities, such as cerebral palsy and intellectual disability. The risk for genetic disorders, such as neural tube defects or GI and cardiac abnormalities, is twice that of single gestations.

Twin pregnancies

Twin pregnancies may be monozygotic (division of the fertilized ovum into two) AKA identical and dizygotic (two separate ova fertilized by two separate sperm) AKA fraternal. Rates of twinning increase markedly with use of fertility agents or assisted reproduction; twins typically deliver at about 37 weeks. Monozygotic twins face extra challenges depending on the point at which the fertilized ovum divided after conception:
- ≤ 3 days - Dichorionic diamniotic membranes: Each fetus is surrounded by a separate amnion and chorion with two separate placentas or one larger placenta for both. This accounts for approximately 20% to 30% of monozygotic twins.
- 4 to 8 days - Monochorionic diamniotic membranes: Each fetus has a separate amnion but one chorion encloses both twins with one placenta. This accounts for approximately 70% to 80% of monozygotic twins.
- 9 to 12 days - Monochorionic monoamniotic membranes: Both fetuses are enclosed in a single amnion and chorion with one placenta. This accounts for 1% of monozygotic twins and has a 50% mortality rate.
- ≥ 12 days - Incomplete division resulting in conjoined twins.

TTTS

With monochorionic gestation and the sharing of one placenta, twin fetuses are at increased risk of twin-to-twin transfusion syndrome (TTTS). With this condition, the blood flow between the twins mixes because of abnormal placental blood vessels with one twin serving as the donor twin and the other the recipient, with severe implications for both:
- Donor twin: Impaired growth, anemia, and hypovolemia
- Recipient twin: Hypertension, polycythemia, CHF, and hypervolemia

Because of the hypervolemia of the recipient twin, this fetus develops increased urinary output, resulting in increased amniotic fluid. The other twin may have oligohydramnios. If they are in separate sacs, the pressure of the increased amniotic fluid in one displaces the other sac resulting in intrauterine growth restriction. TTTS may occur at any point during the pregnancy, even during delivery. Chronic TTTS with onset at 12 to 26 weeks gestation has increased morbidity and mortality because the fetuses may be too immature for delivery. Acute TTTS occurs suddenly, often late in the pregnancy, resulting in increased survival but often with impairments.

Fetal malpresentation

The following are common types of fetal malpresentation:
- Military - The head is erect and neck not flexed, but this poses little problem because flexion often occurs as the head descends.
- Brow - The neck is extended so that the brow presents first. This presentation may relate to SGA, LGA, hydramnios, and uterine or fetal anomalies. Brow presentation, with the largest diameter (about 13.5 cm), increases fetal mortality because of birth trauma, which can include compression of the neck and cerebrum and tracheal and laryngeal damage. Vaginal delivery with episiotomy or cesarean is usually required.
- Face - The neck is severely extended so that the face presents first (about 9.5 cm diameter). This often prolongs labor and may result in increased edema of the fetus and trauma to the neck and internal structures. The neonate usually has bruising in the facial skin.
- Breech - This occurs in 4% of births and is frequently related to early labor and delivery (25% at 25 to 26 weeks gestation). Frank breech (buttocks presentation with legs extended upward) is most common, but single or double footling breech or complete breech (buttocks presentation with legs flexed) can occur. Breech presentation is most common with placenta previa, hydramnios, fetal anomalies, and multiple gestations. Cord prolapse is more likely. Head trauma may occur because molding does not occur, and the head can become entrapped. Mortality and morbidity are reduced with cesarean delivery, especially with low or high fetal weight, hyperextension of neck (> 90 degrees), fetal anomalies, and pelvic disproportion.
- Shoulder - This transverse lie poses extreme risk of uterine rupture. The fetus cannot be delivered, and cesarean delivery is required.
- Compound - Two presenting parts, such as the head and a hand, increasing chances of laceration. With fetal distress or uterine dysfunction, cesarean delivery is required.

Fetal distress

Nonreassuring fetal status (formerly fetal distress) occurs in 5% to 10% of pregnancies. Evaluation requires interpretation of indirect fetal measurements, as well as various risk factors, such as maternal substance abuse and health, laboratory information, fetal size, ultrasound, biophysical profile, and nonstress test. Conditions that affect the uteroplacental unit, which provides nutrients and oxygen to the fetus, may result in nonreassuring fetal status:

- Uteroplacental insufficiency:
  o Placental edema associated with maternal diabetes, hydrops fetalis, or Rh isoimmunization
  o Abruptio placentae and placenta previa
  o Postmaturity
  o IUGR
  o Hyperstimulation of uterus
- Compression of umbilical cord:
  o Umbilical cord prolapse, knot, or entanglement
  o Abnormal insertion or development of umbilical cord
  o Oligohydramnios
- Fetal anomalies/conditions:
  o Maternal or fetal sepsis
  o Congenital anomalies
  o IUGR
  o Prematurity or Postmaturity

Uterine inversion

Uterine inversion can occur if the placenta fails to detach from the uterine wall after delivery or if too much traction is applied to the cord to pull the placenta from the uterus before it is detached. Inversion may result in hemorrhage, hypotension, and shock. Types include

- *Incomplete*: The fundus is soft but the uterus has not descended through the cervix
- *Prolapsed*: The fundus is inverted through the vagina
- *Complete*: The complete uterus is inverted and through the vagina
- *Total*: Both the complete uterus and the vagina are inverted (rare)

Risk factors include prolonged labor, placenta accreta, uterine abnormalities, and short cord. Treatment options include manual reinsertion, surgical reinsertion, hysterectomy, or hydrostatic correction (inflating the vagina with fluid, normal saline, to force the uterus back into position). If the placenta is still attached, it may be removed prior to methods to correct the inversion, but this may increase the danger of hemorrhage; however, leaving the placenta attached may make it more difficult to correct the inversion.

Uterine rupture

Uterine rupture is a rare complication of labor and usually occurs in those having vaginal birth after cesarean, especially those with incisions of the upper uterine segment or fundus (approaching 25% to 33%). Hyperstimulation, sometimes related to *Pitocin* induction, uterine abnormalities, grand multiparity, and obstructed labors (such as with fetal macrosomia or fetopelvic disproportion) are also risk factors. Rupture may occur slowly, leaving the peritoneum intact. In this case, bleeding is minimal and the delivery often proceeds with the tear discovered on postpartum examination. However, with a rapid tear that includes the peritoneum and uterine wall, bleeding is more intense and the fetus may extrude through the uterus with separation of the placenta and nonreassuring fetal status with fetal heart decelerations, bradycardia, or absent fetal heart activity. Treatment is emergency laparotomy, retrieval of the fetus with resuscitation if possible, and repair of the torn tissue. In some cases, hysterectomy may be required.

Premature labor

Preterm or premature labor occurs within weeks 20 to 37. Premature rupture of membrane (PROM) occurs when the membranes rupture before the onset of labor and may lead to premature labor. There are numerous causes for PROM, including infections and digital pelvic exams. When a woman presents in labor, the estimated date of delivery should be obtained by questioning the date of the last menstrual period (LMP) and using a gestation calculator wheel or estimating with Naegele's rule: First day LMP minus 3 months plus 7 days = estimated date of delivery. Fetal viability is very low before 23 weeks of gestation but by 25 weeks, delaying delivery for 2 days can increase survival rates by 10%. Tocolytic drugs, which have many negative adverse effects, may be used to delay delivery in order to administer glucocorticoids, such as betamethasone or dexamethasone, to improve fetal lung maturity between weeks 24 and 36.

Tocolysis

Tocolysis suppresses preterm labor and premature birth, sometimes allowing time to administer betamethasone to accelerate maturity of fetal lungs. Tocolytics (some off-label) include:
- Nifedipine a calcium channel blocker that reduces muscle contractility is most commonly used, as it is more effective and safer than many other drugs. It may increase fetal heart rate (FHR).
- Terbutaline is a beta-adrenergic asthma drug that also relaxes the uterine muscle. It may increase FHR.
- Magnesium sulfate is similar in action to terbutaline, but it requires close monitoring for maternal adverse effects. It crosses the placenta, and the neonate may suffer respiratory and motor depression.
- Indomethacin is an NSAID that inhibits prostaglandin production, and can be used up to 32 weeks of gestation. It crosses the placenta and can cause reduction in amniotic fluid, leading to fetal distress, especially at more than 32 weeks. Indomethacin can also cause premature closure of the ductus arteriosus.
- Ritodrine is a beta-2 adrenergic agonist that relaxes smooth muscles and can delay delivery for 24 to 48 hours but may increase fetal heart rate.

Polyhydramnios

Polyhydramnios is increased amounts of amniotic fluid (more than 500 mL) present during fetal development and is associated with an elevated perinatal mortality rate. Approximately 25% of pregnant women with polyhydramnios experience preterm labor and delivery of a premature infant. Approximately 20% of infants born to mothers with polyhydramnios have an associated anomaly. Some conditions associated with polyhydramnios include:

- Obstructive lesions in the GI tract, such as duodenal atresia or tracheoesophageal fistula with esophageal atresia
- Anencephaly
- Central nervous system anomalies that impair the swallowing reflex
- Cardiovascular rhythm anomalies associated with hydrops
- Twin-to-twin transfusion syndrome in multiple pregnancies
- Macrosomia
- Fetal or neonatal hydrops
- Chromosomal abnormalities such as trisomy 21, 18, or 13
- Skeletal malformations such as congenital hip dislocation, clubfoot, or limb reduction
- Increased risk for prolapsed umbilical cord and placental abruption

Precipitous/precipitate labor

Precipitous/precipitate labor and birth occurs when onset of labor to birth takes only 3 hours or less, often because of strong uterine contractions and low muscle resistance in maternal tissue that promotes rapid dilation of the cervix (or lacerations) and descent of the fetus. A primigravida may dilate 5 cm per hour and a multigravida 10 cm per hour. The neonate may have a low Apgar score and is at increased risk for aspiration of meconium and intracranial injury, such as subdural/dural tears. The strong uterine contractions may interfere with uterine blood flow and oxygenation of the fetus. Precipitous birth alone (without obvious labor), by contrast, is usually an unexpected and sudden birth that takes place outside of the hospital or is unattended by a physician because there is no time to travel or get help. In these cases, the neonate is sometimes expelled into a toilet or onto the floor, causing injury.

Prolonged labor

Prolonged labor results from dysfunctional uterine contractions and is the most common reason for cesarean in nulliparous women, accounting for 50%; only 5% of cesareans are in multiparous women. Dysfunctional contractions are often irregular, exhibit low amplitude, and result in less than 1 cm cervical dilation per hour. In some cases, contractions continue but cervical dilation is arrested. Cesarean may be indicated.

Labor patterns associated with prolonged labor include:
- Hypertonic: Ineffectual contractions in the latent phase of labor become more frequent but do not result in dilation or effacement. The resting tone of the myometrium increases. The contractions may interfere with uteroplacental exchange, resulting in fetal distress. The pressure on the fetal head may result in cephalhematoma, caput succedaneum, or excessive molding. Oxytocin infusion or amniotomy may be used after assessment for cephalopelvic disproportion (CPD).
- Hypotonic: Fewer than 3 contractions in 10 minutes during active phase with less than 1 cm dilatation per hour or arrest of dilatation. Treatment is the same as for hypertonic patterns.

Emergency birth

<u>PROM</u>
Premature rupture of membranes (PROM): The amniotic sac breaks, ideally at term (40 weeks), prior to onset of labor. PROM occurs if labor fails to commence within an hour. About 80% go into labor within 24 hours, and if labor does not commence in 12 to 24 hours, the patient must be frequently monitored until labor begins to ensure adequate amniotic fluid remains, or labor may be induced to prevent infection if the child is at term.

<u>SROM</u>
Spontaneous rupture (SROM): Usually occurs in the early stage of labor during an intense contraction, causing the fluid to gush out of the vagina.

<u>PPROM</u>
Preterm premature rupture of membranes (PPROM): Occurs in a woman less than 37 weeks of gestation and prior to the onset of labor. The patient is monitored as with premature rupture. It is one of the leading causes of premature birth.

<u>PROM</u>
Prolonged rupture of membranes: Prolonged PROM that persists for greater than 18 to 24 hours prior to the onset of labor. It is associated with increased risk of infection in the neonate.

<u>Chorioamnionitis</u>
Chorioamnionitis is an intraamniotic infection caused by bacterial infection of the membranes before delivery. Chorioamnionitis occurs in 3% to 15% of cases of PROM and up to 25% of cases of PPROM. Chorioamnionitis poses a risk of sepsis to both the mother and fetus. The mother usually exhibits fever at least 100.5°F, tachycardia (more than 120 bpm), hypotension, and uterine tenderness. The fetus exhibits tachycardia (160 to 180 bpm). The mother's white blood cell count may be elevated more than 15,000 cell/mcL, and purulent cervical discharge (usually a late sign) may occur. Chorioamnionitis may cause spontaneous onset of labor. Infants are at increased risk of cerebral palsy and early-onset sepsis. The most common pathogenic agents are gram-negative organisms, particularly *Escherichia coli.* Treatment includes intravenous antibiotics and prompt delivery through induction, labor augmentation, or cesarean. The infant must be evaluated at birth and may require treatment for infection as well.

Postterm pregnancy

Postterm pregnancy (more than 294 days or 42 weeks past first day of last menstrual period) occurs in 3% to 7% of pregnancies, and is often the result of errors in calculating due date, but true postterm pregnancies, while posing little risk to the mother, can increase risk to the fetus, and vaginal birth may be facilitated by forceps or vacuum extractor. Increased fetal risks include:
- Large for gestational age (LGA) more than 4,500 g (about 10 pounds), which may result in prolonged labor, birth trauma with fractures or neurological injury, or cesarean delivery
- Aspiration of meconium occurs more frequently because a large fetus is more likely to expel meconium

- Postmaturity syndrome related to restriction of growth in the uterus, often because of restricted blood flow, putting the fetus at risk for respiratory and neurological disorders

Oligohydramnios

Oligohydramnios is decreased amounts of amniotic fluid (less than 500 mL). Amniotic fluid cushions the fetus during development and is also necessary for normal development of the lungs. After 20 weeks of gestation, amniotic fluid is mainly produced by the fetus's excretion of urine. Fluids secreted by the respiratory tract and the oral/nasal cavity also contribute to the production of amniotic fluid. Oligohydramnios signals significant congenital pathology in the fetus and is associated with an elevated perinatal mortality rate. Some conditions associated with oligohydramnios include:
- Urinary tract anomalies:
  o Obstructive uropathy
  o Renal agenesis
  o Polycystic kidneys
- Pulmonary hypoplasia
- Pressure deformities, such as clubbed feet
- Compression of the umbilical cord, leading to fetal hypoxia
- Meconium staining
- Postterm gestation
- Leaking of amniotic fluid or prolonged or premature rupture of membranes, which are risk factors for neonatal infections

Dependence on drugs

The mother who has dependence on drugs poses considerable problems during labor, with increased risk to both the mother and the fetus. If the mother begins labor and is currently using illicit drugs, she may be uncooperative, drug seeking, lethargic, or hyperactive, depending on the substance. She may be in danger of developing withdrawal symptoms, which increase risk to the fetus. Drug addicts typically have increased risk of infections, such as hepatitis, HIV/AIDS, and other sexually transmitted diseases. Ideally, the mother's dependence was identified prior to labor and the mother maintained with either methadone or buprenorphine, which can prevent withdrawal and pose a lower risk to the fetus. Both treatments require careful and ongoing monitoring to ensure compliance after a period of stabilization (usually 2 to 3 days). During labor and delivery, those women maintained on methadone or buprenorphine should use those drugs for pain control, with careful monitoring to avoid overmedicating.

Amphetamines

Amphetamines are a class of drugs that cause CNS stimulation. The most commonly abused amphetamine is methamphetamine. Maternal use of these substances causes hypertension and tachycardia, which can cause miscarriage, abruptio placentae, and premature delivery. Vasoconstriction affects placental vessels, decreasing circulation, nutrition, and oxygen to the fetus. Additionally, users often have depressed appetite and may have malnutrition. Methamphetamines can cross the placental barrier and cause fetal hypertension and prenatal strokes and damage to the heart and other organs. The neonate is commonly small for gestational age, often 5 pounds or less, or full-term but 10th percentile or less for weight, with shortened length and smaller head circumference. The neonate in withdrawal from maternal amphetamine use will suffer abnormal sleep patterns, often characterized by lethargy and excessive sleeping during the first few weeks, poor feeding, tremors, diaphoresis, miosis, frantic fist sucking, high-pitched crying, fever, excessive yawning, and hyperreflexia.

Cocaine/crack

Cocaine/crack (freebase cocaine) is a nonopioid substance that readily crosses the placenta through simple diffusion. One of the most potent properties of cocaine is its ability to act as a vasoconstrictor. When a mother uses cocaine the blood supply to the placenta is severely compromised when the vessels constrict, compromising blood flow and resulting in growth retardation and hypoxia. Cocaine also causes a programmed cell death (known as apoptosis) in the heart muscle cells of the fetus, resulting in cardiac dysfunction for the fetus. Maternal cocaine use increases the risk of premature birth and causes serious consequences for the neonate after birth, including cerebral infarctions, nonduodenal intestinal atresia, anal atresia, necrotizing enterocolitis (NEC), defects of the limbs, and genitourinary defects. Cocaine stimulates the central nervous system by limiting the uptake of certain neurotransmitters such as norepinephrine, serotonin, and dopamine. Cocaine has a direct toxic effect on the fetal nervous system, so the infant will exhibit extreme irritability and tremors followed by sluggish, lethargic behavior.

Heroin

Heroin, an illegal opioid narcotic, is highly addictive. Users are at increased risk of HIV/AIDS from sharing needles, as well as cellulitis, endocarditis, and abscesses. Pregnant users may experience poor nutrition, iron deficiency anemia, and preeclampsia-eclampsia, all negatively affecting the fetus. Premature birth, early placental separation, and breech presentation are common. If the mother tries to stop using heroin, she may go into withdrawal, which can trigger premature labor, spontaneous abortion, or stillbirth. Symptoms of withdrawal usually start within 12 hours and include agitation, insomnia, increased sweating, and runny nose, progressing to gastrointestinal effects that include cramping, diarrhea, nausea, and vomiting. Pregnant women may be placed on a program of methadone maintenance under careful medical supervision because methadone, while posing less danger to the fetus, is also addictive. However, methadone may delay withdrawal symptoms and reduce cravings. Additionally, while neonates may exhibit jitteriness, fever, poor feeding, and vomiting after birth, the symptoms are usually transient.

Methadone

Methadone is commonly used to treat women who are addicted to heroin because it blocks withdrawal symptoms and drug craving, but methadone crosses the placental barrier and exposes the fetus to the drug. Many female heroin users are of reproductive age, and methadone is often administered to pregnant women to decrease dangers associated with heroin, such as fluctuating levels of drug and exposure to hepatitis and HIV from sharing of needles. Exposure to methadone may result in miscarriage, stillbirth, intrauterine growth restriction, fetal distress, and low birth rate, although symptoms are usually less severe than with heroin. However, if the mother takes methadone along with other drugs, this can compound the adverse effects. Additionally, sudden withdrawal from methadone may cause preterm labor or death of the fetus, so methadone should be monitored carefully.

Induction of labor

Induction of labor stimulates uterine contractions to speed birth and may be done for many conditions, including diabetes mellitus, preeclampsia, postterm gestation, mild abruptio placentae, oligohydramnios, and poor biophysical profile. Induction is contraindicated with abnormal fetal heart rate patters, breech or uncertain presentation, multiple gestation, maternal heart disease or hypertension, and polyhydramnios. Common induction methods include:
- Stripping/sweeping amniotic membrane: A gloved finger is inserted through the cervical os and rotated (360 degrees) twice to separate the amniotic membrane from the lower part of the uterus in order to release prostaglandins and stimulate contractions. Although not always effective, labor usually begins in 24 to 48 hours.
- Oxytocin infusion: Oxytocin (*Pitocin*) is used to stimulate contractions of the uterus for induction of labor, but risks include overstimulating the uterus, causing too frequent/intense contractions, and uterine rupture and water intoxication.
- Complementary methods: These methods include sexual intercourse, nipple stimulation, and herbal/homeopathic preparations. These methods have few negative effects.

Cesarean deliveries

Cesarean deliveries are done if there is increased risk of uterine rupture, maternal hemorrhage, dystocia including fetal-pelvic disproportion and breech presentation, active herpes infection, and emergent situations, such as fetal distress or impending maternal death. Regional anesthesia (spinal, epidural) is associated with lower mortality than general anesthesia, so it is the preferred anesthetic approach. Additionally, there is less fetal depression, reduced risk of maternal pulmonary aspiration, and an opportunity to provide neuraxial analgesia for postoperative pain relief. Regional anesthesia must provide a T4 sensory level, which causes a high sympathetic blockade. In some cases, general anesthesia may be administered for cesarean delivery, although the risks to the mother are intensified, so general anesthesia is usually limited to emergent situations in which the mother or fetus are at risk:
- Fetal distress during second stage of labor
- Tetanic uterine contractions
- Patient confused and uncontrollable and unable to cooperate (such as psychiatric patients)
- Inverted uterus
- Retained placenta
- Breech extraction or other position requiring version and extraction.

Prolapsed umbilical cord

A prolapse of the umbilical cord occurs when the umbilical cord precedes the fetus in the birth canal and becomes entrapped by the descending fetus. An occult cord prolapse occurs when the umbilical cord is beside or just ahead of the fetal head. About half of prolapses occur in the second stage of labor and relate to premature delivery, multiple gestation, polyhydramnios, breech delivery, and an excessively long umbilical cord. Some cases are precipitated by obstetric interventions, such as amniotomy, external eversion, and application of scalp electrode for monitoring. As contractions occur and the head descends, this applies pressure to the umbilical cord, occluding blood flow and causing hypoxia and bradycardia. The decrease in blood flow through the umbilical vessels can cause impaired gas exchange, and if pressure on the cord is not relieved, the fetus can suffer severe neurological damage or death. Management includes elevating the presenting part off the cord, having the mother elevate her knees to the chest, and preparing for cesarean delivery.

Pregnancy and bleeding disorders

Mothers with bleeding disorders (von Willebrand disease, hemophilia A or B, factor XI deficiency) require careful monitoring during pregnancy and factor levels kept within normal limits because of increased risk of hemorrhage during labor and delivery. While vaginal birth is not contraindicated, prolonged labor should be avoided. Blood samples should be obtained at onset of labor for blood cell counts and clotting panels with planning based on factor levels during the last trimester. If levels have been low, the mother may receive prophylactic factor infusion, usually with recombinant products, if possible, to decrease risk of viral transmission to the fetus. Desmopressin may be used to increase factor VIII and VWF, although this requires careful monitoring because of possibility of fluid overload. Regional anesthesia may be used if clotting levels are within normal range but poses increased risk of bleeding with low levels. Invasive fetal monitoring is contraindicated if the fetus is at risk for inheriting the bleeding disorder, and a cord blood sample should be obtained for evaluation immediately after birth.

Delivery

Spinal anesthesia

A saddle block, or spinal anesthesia, is usually given just before vaginal delivery to provide rapid perineal anesthesia. Spinal blocks are avoided during labor because they interfere with motor function. Because of this, other agents may be used during labor. Prior to receiving the spinal anesthesia, the patient is given a bolus of 500 to 1,000 mL fluid. With the patient in sitting position, a very small spinal needle (to prevent CSF leakage and postspinal headache) is inserted into the subarachnoid space. Local anesthetics used include hyperbaric tetracaine, bupivacaine, or lidocaine, often with the addition of fentanyl or sufentanil to potentiate the effect. The agents are administered between contractions over about 30 seconds. The patient remains sitting for 3 minutes and then is placed in lithotomy position with left uterine displacement to prepare for delivery.

Expulsive period

During the expulsive period of delivery, the mother will need to be coached so as to achieve effective pushing effort. Two types of pushing are effective: Open-glottis physiological pushing, and closed-glottis (Valsalva) pushing. The mother should be coached on the method most effective for her. During crowning, the mother should be instructed to "pant like a puppy." The integrity of the perineum needs to be taken into consideration. Most mothers would like to avoid an episiotomy if at all possible; however, there are several factors that may require episiotomy:
- Fetal malposition
- Anticipation of the delivery of a large baby
- Possibility of shoulder dystocia (where the anterior shoulder cannot pass below the symphysis pubis)
- Poor elasticity of the perineal tissue
- Difficulty in maintaining adequate control of the patient's expulsive efforts

Placenta

The placenta will generally deliver 5 to 30 minutes after delivery of the fetus. The mechanism of placental separation starts with the change in the size of the uterus, and then proceeds by the formation of a hematoma between the placenta and uterine wall, the separation of the placenta, the descent of the placenta through the lower uterine segment and vagina, and then expulsion. Signs and symptoms of placental separation include a sudden increase in vaginal bleeding, lengthening of the umbilical cord, and the rising of the uterus in the abdomen. Management of placental delivery includes obtaining cord blood samples after the cord is clamped, inspecting the cord for the number of vessels, and avoiding uterine massage and cord traction until the placenta is separated. Pushing by the mother may assist in expulsion of the placenta. If membranes follow the placenta, hold the placenta and roll over and over until the membranes are delivered.

Placental abnormalities/variations

The following are types of placental abnormalities/variations:
- Battledore - Cord is attached at the periphery of the placenta, usually of no clinical concern. Occurs in up to one-third of twin pregnancies.
- Succenturiate lobed - An accessory placenta is within the fetal sac and maintains vascular connections with the main placenta, sometimes resulting in retained placental tissue or hemorrhage, especially if large.
- Velamentous cord insertion - Cord inserts into the membranes rather than the middle of the placenta, traveling through the chorion and amnion to reach the placenta, leaving exposed unprotected vessels. This can cause shearing of the blood vessels during delivery, leading to hemorrhage.
- Circumvallate - A fibrous band of tissue, caused by a double layer of chorion and amnion, appears on the fetal side of the placenta, resulting in deep implantation, but is usual of no clinical concern.

Birthing positions

The different birthing positions are explained as follows:
- Hands and knees:
    - Increases perineal relaxation, reducing lacerations and need for episiotomy, and facilitating birth with shoulder dystocia.
    - Improves circulation to placenta and umbilical cord.
    - Relieves discomfort of "back labor" but may be fatiguing.
    - Prevents face-to-face contact with mother.
    - Prevents use of instruments, so positional change sometimes required, and prevents mother from viewing birth.
    - Comfort measures: Provide pillows for support under chest and upper thighs.
- Left lateral Sims':
    - Increases perineal relaxation, reducing need for episiotomy.
    - Prevents compromise of peripheral venous return.
    - Slows fetal descent and reduces danger of aspiration.
    - Prevents mother from viewing birth.
    - Increases comfort, but requires repositioning if forceps needed or for repair of episiotomy.
    - Comfort measures: Position mother so that upper leg is supported by pillows, the bed, or partner.
- Semi-Fowler's:
    - Prevents compromise of peripheral venous return.
    - Allows mother to view birth. Decreases perineal relaxation if legs are spread widely.
    - Does not make use of gravity assist, so often used in later stages of labor. Increases mother's comfort level, especially for long labors.
    - Comfort measures: Provide adequate support for upper body, legs, and feet using pillows and changing bed position.
- Sitting (birthing bed):
    - Speeds fetal descent because of pull of gravity.
    - Prevents compromise of peripheral venous return.
    - Allows mother to change leg positions and view birth. Allows a supported sitting position.
    - Comfort measures: Provide adequate support for lower extremities.
- Sitting (birthing chair/Stool):
    - Speeds fetal descent and delivery, reducing need for operative procedures.
    - Prevents compromise of peripheral venous return. Allows mother to view birth.
    - Prevents back support (stool), but reduces pain of "back labor." Comfort measures: Allow mother to change position to increase comfort.
- Squatting:
    - Increases pelvic outlet, speeding fetal descent and delivery.
    - May shorten second stage of labor.
    - Decreases attendant's view of and access to perineum.
    - Increases difficulty of monitoring fetal status and instrument use and increases perineal edema.

- o Comfort measures: Provide birthing bar for mother to hold onto and balance support.
- Recumbent:
  - o Allows maintenance of sterile field, good access and view of perineum, and ease of episiotomy.
  - o Decreases maternal blood pressure.
  - o Increases pressure on diaphragm and maternal dyspnea. Increases risk of laceration and need for episiotomy. Increases risk of aspiration.
  - o May interfere with intensity and frequency of uterine contractions, and increases maternal discomfort. Allows mother to view birth.
  - o Comfort measures: Avoid use of stirrups if possible or ensure they are not causing pressure on lower extremities.
  - o Monitor circulation and provide support for legs.

Forceps-assisted birth

Forceps-assisted birth uses a variety of specialized tools to assist with the birth of the fetus by providing traction and a method of rotating the fetal head into proper occiput-anterior position. Most forceps are used with the fetus in head down position and the forceps positioned on the sides of the head:

- Outlet forceps application can be used when the perineum is bulging, scalp is visible between contractions, or the sagittal suture is not more than 45 degrees from midline. The fetal skull must be at station +2 or below
- Midforceps application requires the head be engaged but the leading edge above +2 station
- High forceps are no longer used

Indications for forceps-assisted birth include conditions that pose a risk to the mother or fetus and are relieved by birth. Maternal risks of forceps-assisted birth include infection, cervical and birth canal lacerations, extension of episiotomy, anal sphincter injury, and weakening of pelvic floor muscles. Neonatal risks include bruising and edema of face, caput succedaneum, cephalhematoma, transient low Apgar score, retinal hemorrhage, ocular trauma, Erb palsy, and elevated bilirubin.

Vacuum-assisted birth

Vacuum-assisted birth utilizes a soft suction cup attached to a suction pump that creates negative pressure of 50 to 60 mm Hg. The suction cup is applied to the occiput of the fetus and traction is applied with contractions. Suction use should be limited to 20 to 30 minutes, with scalp trauma more likely after 10 minutes of use. If the suction cup dislodges more than 3 times, use should be discontinued. Indications include prolonged second stage of labor or nonreassuring heart pattern. Vacuum-assisted birth may also be used if the mother is too fatigued to push. Neonatal risks include scalp lacerations, subdural hematoma, cephalhematoma, intracranial hemorrhage, subconjunctival hemorrhage, Erb palsy, 6th and 9th cranial nerve trauma, retinal hemorrhage, and death. A caput forms on the neonate's head, but should subside in 2 to 3 days. Maternal risks include perineal trauma, lacerations, pain, and infection.

Cesarean birth

Cesarean births have a higher mortality rate than vaginal births, with complications including infection, blood clots, and hemorrhage. The cesarean is usually done with a regional (spinal, epidural) anesthetic rather than general anesthetic because general anesthesia poses more risks to the mother and causes more fetal depression. Regional anesthesia must provide a T4 sensory level (high sympathetic blockade). An opioid and nitrous oxide or propofol may be administered after the delivery is complete to provide amnesia and prevent recall. If the mother was nonfasting or aspiration is a concern, an orogastric tube may be inserted and aspiration of stomach contents done to reduce the chance of aspiration during emergence from general anesthesia. Additionally, the patient should be extubated only after awake. Blood loss with cesarean delivery is about 1,000 mL, so fluid replacement must balance estimated loss.

Skin and uterine incisions

Cesarean births require two different types of incisions. Skin incisions may be transverse or vertical. Transverse incisions leave less obvious scarring but delivery takes longer. Likewise, uterine incisions may be vertical or transverse, but not always the same as the skin incision:
- Kerr incision: The most common uterine incision is the transverse lower uterine incision because the uterus is thinnest, bleeding is less, repair is easier, adhesion development is less, bladder dissection is less, and risk of rupture with subsequent pregnancies decreases; however, the size is restricted by major vessels on the sides, and the incision requires more time.
- Sellheim incision: Vertical incision in the lower uterus is usually used for multiple gestation, malpresentation, placenta previa, macrosomia, and preterm deliveries because it allows better access and faster delivery, but this approach carries a greater risk of rupture with subsequent pregnancies (which then require cesarean delivery), and requires more dissection of the bladder.

Neonate care

This neonate's transition period begins immediately after the delivery when the infant stabilizes and adjusts to life outside of the womb. This involves three stages: the first period of reactivity, the period of unresponsive sleep, and the second period of reactivity; however, these stages may undergo alteration if there is significant stress during labor and/or delivery. To minimize stress to the infant, contact with the mother should be maintained, and examinations and/or procedures should be delayed if appropriate. The neonate's transition to life occurs in three stages:
- First period of reactivity - This period begins immediately after delivery and lasts about 30 minutes. Assessment should show heartbeat and respirations near the upper limits of normal, respiratory rales for about 20 minutes, alertness, the startle reflex, and crying. Breastfeeding should be encouraged during this period as it helps the blood glucose level to drop to normal within 90 minutes after delivery.
- Period of unresponsive sleep - This period occurs after the first period of reactivity and lasts from 30 minutes after birth to 2 hours after birth. During this period, the heart rate decreases to less than 140 bpm, a heart murmur may be present because of incomplete closure of the ductus arteriosus, and the respirations are slow and become more regular.

- Second period of reactivity - This period lasts from 2 to 6 hours after birth. During this time, the heart rate may become unstable and changing, there may be rapid changes in skin color, and the respirations slow to less than 60 per minute; however, the rales should clear by this time. The infant may be interested in feeding, which will help prevent hypoglycemia, stimulate a bowel movement, and prevent jaundice.

Rapid assessment

The infant should be given a rapid assessment within seconds of birth to determine if the infant is at term, if the amniotic fluid is clear, if there is muscle tone, and if there are respirations or crying. If any of these conditions are not met, then the neonate should be placed under radiant heat and further resuscitation done. The basic steps to resuscitation include:
- Warming the infant after drying
- Positioning the infant and clearing the airway if necessary
- Stimulating and repositioning the infant

The infant should be evaluated throughout the initial procedures:
- Respirations: Rate and character of respirations should be noted as well as observation of chest wall movement
- Heart rate: Should be more than 100 bpm, assessed with stethoscope or at the base of the umbilical cord

Neonatal assessment

The neonate should undergo three different types of physical assessment:
- Immediate: The first examination is done in the delivery room to determine the need for resuscitation or other intervention. This includes Apgar assessment
- 1 to 4 hours after birth: The second examination includes gestational age assessment, which must be completed within 24 hours for accuracy, and brief physical assessment to determine if there are any problems that might place the infant at risk. This includes assessment of respiratory and cardiac status, cord color, skin color, and movement. The Modified Ballard scoring system is often used
- At least 24 hours after birth (or prior to discharge): The final examination should include a complete physical and behavioral assessment that includes all systems and evaluation of reflexes. All weights and measurements are taken and reviewed. This exam requires observation, palpation, and auscultation. In some cases, instead of a separate examination at 1 to 4 hours, only this complete physical examination is done

Providing warmth

Infants have poor temperature regulation ability, particularly preterm infants who lack brown fat, which is one of the body's tools to regulate body temperature. Providing warmth is critical as a component of resuscitation. An infant who is just seconds old and wet will need aggressive measures to keep it warm while any resuscitation efforts are being initiated. Infants lose heat through their head so one of the first steps should be to place a hat on the head. The infant should be placed under a radiant heater and vigorous drying with warmed blankets should begin. Often this stimulation, drying and warming, is all that is needed to establish a regular respiration pattern in the neonate. Preterm infants weighing less than 1,500 g should be placed in a plastic bag (made specifically for this purpose) up to the height of the shoulders to prevent cold shock. A term infant with no apparent distress can be placed on the mother's chest and covered with a warm blanket.

APGAR delivery room assessment

Dr. Virginia Apgar developed the APGAR test in 1952. APGAR stands for Appearance, Pulse, Grimace, Activity, and Respiration. The APGAR is the first test given to a newborn. It is used as a quick evaluation of a newborn's physical condition to determine if any emergency medical care is needed and is administered 1 minute and 5 minutes after birth. The test is administered more than once, as the baby's condition may change rapidly. It may be administered for a third time 10 minutes after birth if needed. The baby is rated on the five subscales and the scores are added together. A total score of at least 7 is a sign of good health:

- Appearance (skin color):
    - 0 - Cyanotic or pallor over entire body
    - 1 - Normal, except for extremities
    - 2 - Entire body normal
- Pulse (heart rate):
    - 0 – Absent
    - 1 - < 100 bpm
    - 2 - >100 bpm
- Grimace (reflex irritability):
    - 0 – Unresponsive
    - 1 – Grimace
    - 2 - Infant sneezes, coughs, and recoils
- Activity (muscle tone):
    - 0 – Absent
    - 1 - Flexed limbs
    - 2 - Infant moves freely
- Respiration (breathing rate and effort):
    - 0 – Absent
    - 1 - Bradypnea, dyspnea
    - 2 - Good breathing and crying

Cord blood gas interpretation

Umbilical cord blood gas testing, preferably arterial, should be done 60 minutes or less after birth for infants who are at risk or depressed to determine pH and acid-base balance. Testing is most applicable to infants with low APGAR scores (0 to 3) persisting for at least 5 minutes. A pH of less than 7 may indicate birth asphyxia/hypoxia severe enough to cause neurological deficits. Infants with normal APGAR scores may also have pH less than 7 but without pathology, so results must be evaluated in relation to the APGAR scores and child's general condition. Preterm infants often have low APGAR scores and may be suspected of having birth asphyxia, but if they have suffered no birth asphyxia or hypoxia, the pH level usually remains normal.

Normal cord blood values are as follows:
- Venous:
    - pH - 7.25 to 7.35
    - pO_2 - 28 to 32 mm Hg
    - PCO_2 - 40 to 50 mm Hg
    - Base excess - 0 to 5 mEq/L
- Arterial:
    - pH - 7.28
    - pO_2 - 16 to 20 mm Hg
    - PCO_2 - 40 to 50 mm Hg
    - Base excess - 0 to 10 mEq/L

Abnormal cord blood values are as follows:
- Respiratory Acidosis:
    - pH - < 7.25
    - pO_2 - Varies
    - PCO_2 - > 50 mm Hg
    - Base excess - < 10 mEq/L
- Metabolic acidosis:
    - pH - < 7.25
    - pO_2 - < 20 mm Hg
    - PCO_2 - 44 to 55 mm Hg
    - Base excess - > 10 mEq/L

ABCs of infant resuscitation

The ABCs of resuscitation are a device to help remember the order to do which steps of the resuscitation process. In this device, the letters stand for as follows:
- A is Airway - An airway should be established as the very first thing tended to; if there is no airway, air cannot be moved during resuscitation attempts. This step includes clearing the mouth and nose of secretions, and properly positioning the infant in the "sniff" position.
- B is Breathing - This step involves initiating breathing after the airway has been established; this can be done with stimulation, supplemental oxygen, or artificial ventilation.
- C is Circulation - Once an airway and breathing have been established, then the circulation is considered; chest compressions may be indicated here or the administration of volume expanders and possibly epinephrine.

Meconium in amniotic fluid

When meconium is present in the amniotic fluid, the following steps should be taken immediately following birth to avoid meconium aspiration syndrome:
- If the infant is crying and showing no signs of distress, the mouth, nose and throat should be suctioned with a suction catheter and the usual steps of drying and stimulation completed

- If the infant shows signs of respiratory distress in the presence of meconium-stained fluid, the infant should be immediately intubated with an endotracheal tube for the purpose of suctioning the trachea. Once intubated, the trachea can be suctioned with a large catheter attached to wall suction

Once the airway has been adequately suctioned and cleared, the stomach may need to be suctioned as well in order to prevent the regurgitation of the swallowed meconium. Meconium that is swallowed and then regurgitated can be aspirated into the lungs.

Establishing an airway

To establish an airway, the infant is placed supine with the head slightly extended in the "sniffing" position. A small neck roll may be placed under the shoulders to maintain this position in a very small premature infant. Once the proper position is established, the mouth and nose are suctioned (mouth first to prevent reflex inspiration of secretions when nose suctioned) with a bulb syringe or catheter if necessary. The infant's head can be turned momentarily to the side to allow secretions to pool in the cheek where they can be more easily suctioned and removed to establish the airway. Stimulating the newborn is often all that is needed to initiate spontaneous respirations in the neonate. This tactile stimulation can be accomplished by gently rubbing the back or trunk of the infant. Another technique used to provide stimulation is flicking or rubbing the soles of the feet. Slapping neonates as stimulation is no longer practiced and should NOT be used.

Facilitating the attachment progress

Facilitating the attachment process begins before delivery by educating the mother about bonding and the importance of early and close contact with her infant. Ensuring skin-to-skin contact within the first hour is especially important, but different approaches are used:
- If the neonate appears stable at delivery, he/she should be placed on the mother's abdomen for drying and initial assessment and then placed between the mother's breasts and covered with a blanket to prevent temperature loss. Weighing, measuring, and bathing the infant is deferred
- The neonate may be assessed in a warmer, dried, diapered, weighed, and measured and then placed between the mother's breasts
- After delivery, the neonate should be held with skin-to-skin contact as soon as possible and as often as possible

If the mother is breastfeeding, the neonate should start breastfeeding within 30 to 60 minutes of delivery.

Cesarean initial assessments

The initial assessments of the mother who has had a cesarean and the neonate are similar to vaginal birth, but the mother also must recover from a surgical procedure and anesthesia. Immediate postoperative care during the first postpartal hour includes:
- VS are checked every 5 minutes until stable, then every 15 minutes for 1 hour, and finally every 30 minutes until released from the recovery area

- Abdominal dressing and perineal pad should be checked every 15 minutes for bleeding for the first hour and fundus gently palpated with a hand supporting the incisional area
- IV oxytocin is administered to promote contraction of the uterine muscles
- General anesthesia: Patient positioned on side and turned every 2 hours for 24 hours
- Epidural or spinal anesthesia: Level of anesthesia checked every 15 minutes
- Intake and output are monitored and urine checked for signs of blood (indicating bladder trauma)
- Analgesia is given as indicated to control pain

Vaginal birth assessments

During the first postpartal hour, maternal monitoring includes the following assessments:
- Vital signs:
  o VS should be checked every 15 minutes and evaluated in relation to baseline VS and VS prior to delivery
  o Normal BP varies 90 to 140/60 to 90
  o Falling BP and increased pulse may indicate uterine bleeding
  o Pulse (60 to 90) is usually slightly decreased from that found during labor
  o Respirations should be relaxed and not labored, usually ranging 12 to 20/min
- Temperature: Slight elevation is normal immediately after delivery (100.4°F or less) but this should return to normal by 24 hours
- Alertness: The mother should be awake, alert, and responsive, and able to hold infant.
- Fundus:
  o Fundus is palpated to determine if it is firm, midline, and in the expected position (umbilicus)
  o A boggy fundus may indicate uterine bleeding
  o Bladder distention may cause fundus to deviate from midline
- Lochia:
  o Lochia should be checked every 15 minutes for signs of excess bleeding, such as copious discharge or large clots
  o Lochia must be observed while fundus is massaged to determine if there is free flow of blood or expulsion of clots, which may indicate hemorrhage
  o Lochia rubra should be present with moderate amount of discharge, less than 1 perineal pad/hour
- Perineum:
  o Perineal area should be examined and amount of swelling and bruising noted, as well as condition of episiotomy (if present) and sutures
  o Severe perineal/rectal pain requires further examination
- Bladder:
  o The bladder should be palpated to determine if it is distended
  o The mother should be given the opportunity to urinate within the first hour after delivery before catheterization is considered
  o Mother should spontaneously urinate >100 mL clear urine with no distention noted after urination

- Rectum:
  o Rectum should be examined for presence of tearing or hemorrhoids
  o No severe rectal pain should be present
  o If hemorrhoids are present, engorgement must be reported to physician, especially if $\geq$ 2 cm in size
- Pain:
  o Mother should have only mild pain, < 3 on 1 to 10 scale
  o Severe pain requires further examination to determine cause.
  o Analgesia should be provided to control pain
- Legs/feet:
  o Feet and legs should be warm and pulses palpable.
  o Edema, which may have been present before delivery, should remain stable or decrease
- Anesthesia: If the mother had an anesthetic, such as epidural or spinal, the level of anesthesia should be assessed every 15 minutes

Postpartal comfort measures

The mother undergoes multiple physiological changes during the puerperium (postpartal period), beginning immediately after birth, but many of the changes may be alleviated by simple comfort measures:
- Hunger - Mothers often feel very hungry after giving birth and may enjoy a light meal. If the mother had a cesarean delivery, she may be limited to clear liquids initially but should be progressed to a regular diet as soon as possible.
- Thirst - Because fluids are lost during delivery, the mother often experiences marked thirst, alleviated by providing ample oral fluids to replace those lost. If the mother had a cesarean delivery and is receiving IVs, then the rate of replacement must be adequate.
- Chill - Postpartal chill immediately after delivery is common and may relate to neurological or vasomotor changes. The mother should be covered with a warmed blanket and offered warm liquids.
- Diaphoresis - Perspiration increases during the puerperium to help eliminate excess fluid and waste products, but the mother may wake up drenched in sweat at night. The mother should be provided dry gown and linens and protected from chilling.
- Afterpains - With a first pregnancy, the uterus usually remains contracted after delivery, but with sub-sequent pregnancies or complications, such as hydramnios or retention of clots or placental tissue, the uterus may alternate between contraction and relaxation, causing severe cramp-like afterpains in the 2 to 3 days after delivery. Additionally, if the mother receives oxytocin to stimulate contractions, this may increase discomfort. Breastfeeding naturally stimulates release of oxytocin, so breastfeeding may cause afterpains. Analgesic agents, such as acetaminophen or ibuprofen, especially an hour before breast-feeding and at bedtime, may relieve discomfort.
- Flatulence - The GI tract is sluggish after birth because of hormonal changes and decreased muscle tone. Flatulence is common, especially after cesarean delivery. This is alleviated by early ambulation, turning from side to side, avoiding carbonated beverages, and taking antiflatulent medications.

Postpartal Period

Physical Needs of the Mother

Postpartal uterine involution

The normal uterus weighs about 70 to 100 g with a capacity of 5 mL. During pregnancy, the uterus increases in weight to 1,000 g with capacity of 5,000 mL. After delivery, the uterus weight decreases to 500 g by the end of the first week, 300 by the second, and 100 by the third. Uterine involution (the process of the uterus returning to the prepregnant state) begins immediately after the placenta separates. A number of changes occur over the first 3 weeks (except for the placental site, which takes 6 to 7 weeks to heal over):
- Estrogen and progesterone levels drop markedly, causing cells to atrophy and reversing hyperplasia
- Autolysis occurs as proteolytic enzymes are released and macrophages migrate to the uterus.
- The spongy layer of decidua sloughs off as lochia
- The basal layer of decidua separates into two layers within 48 to 72 hours with the outer layer becoming necrotic and sloughing off as lochia and the inner layer providing the base for the new endometrium

Fundus postpartal evaluation

The uterus contracts after the placenta is expelled to about grapefruit size with the fundus about midway to two-thirds the distance between the symphysis pubis and the umbilicus. The contraction of the uterus brings the uterine walls together and compresses the vessels to prevent bleeding:
- Over the 6 to 12 hours after delivery, blood and clots pool in the uterus, and the fundus rises midline to the level of the umbilicus, where it stays for about 12 hours. A fundus above the umbilicus and boggy indicates excessive bleeding. A high fundus that deviates from midline often indicates a distended bladder
- By first postpartum day, the fundus is about 1 cm (one finger-width) below the umbilicus
- The fundus continues to descend about 1 cm per day until it is no longer palpable (usually within 2 weeks)

If a boggy uterus is felt on fundal examination, it should be massaged until the uterus contracts, expels clots and debris, and firms. If it fails to firm, the physician should be notified

Lochia assessment

Lochia, vaginal discharge after delivery, rids the uterus of remaining debris. The total volume of discharge is about 240 to 480 mL, with discharge decreasing over time. Discharge is usually increased in the morning because of pooling. Lochia should be examined to assess both hemorrhage and uterine involution:

- Rubra - Days 1 to 3 or 4. Dark red discharge, containing epithelial cells, red and white blood cells, bacteria, decidua shreds, lanugo, vernix caseosa, and sometimes meconium. Clots should not exceed nickel size, large clots may indicate hemorrhage, this should be differentiated from bleeding from vaginal lacerations.
- Serosa - Days 4 to 10. Pinkish to brownish discharge, containing serous exudate, decidua shreds, red and white blood cells, cervical mucus, and various microorganisms. Lightens as number of red blood cells decrease.
- Alba - Persists additional 2 to 85 days (average 24). Yellowish discharge contains primarily white blood cells, epithelial cells, decidual cells, fat, mucus, and bacteria. The cervix is closed when lochia alba flow stops, so the danger of infection ceases.

Breasts postpartal assessment

Hormonal changes with birth stimulate the breasts to increase milk production. The mother may feel some increased fullness. The breasts should feel full but not hard on gentle palpation and may be slightly tender. The mother should be advised to avoid sleeping in the prone position, as this compresses the breasts and increases the risk of complications, such as clogged milk duct. Breastfeeding should begin immediately or within 30 to 60 minutes of birth. Colostrum does not pose a danger to the neonate, even if aspirated, and breastfeeding promotes bonding with the infant and contraction of the uterus. Colostrum, produced the first 2 to 4 days, is thick and yellow and produced only in teaspoons, but this is adequate for the neonate whose stomach capacity the first day is only 5 to 7 mL. Colostrum provides both antibodies and protein. By day 3, transitional milk is thinning, and the stomach capacity is 1 ounce. By day 7, when mature milk is starting to come in, the neonate's stomach capacity is 1.5 to 2 ounces.

Psychosocial and Health Needs of the Family

Maternal/newborn separation

Maternal/Newborn separation should be avoided as much as possible as it interferes with the bonding and causes distress to the neonate. In some cases, such as with cesarean delivery or premature birth, some separation is necessary but nursing staff should facilitate contact. Babies who are held with skin-to-skin contact often cry less and breastfeed better. In many facilities, immediate skin-to-skin contact occurs after vaginal and cesarean delivery, with the mother encouraged to hold and breastfeed the child during the initial assessment. Mothers should be encouraged to utilize rooming and should be with their babies at all times for the first few days as this facilitates bonding and helps the mother learn to recognize the babies cues. Additionally, mothers who room in around the clock are more likely to breastfeed exclusively rather than resorting to supplementary bottle feedings.

Maternal attachment process

By the time of birth, most mothers have developed an emotional connection with her infant and demonstrate a number of typical steps in the maternal attachment process:
- Touching: The mother usually begins by lightly touching the infant's extremities with her fingertips and moving toward running the palm over the baby's trunk. This exploration of the infant can proceed very quickly (minutes) or be more tentative and take days. Early skin-to-skin contact with the infant tends to accelerate this process.
- En face positioning: The mother increases the amount of face-to-face eye contact with the infant, typically holding the infant close to her face and responding to eye contact by speaking in a sing-song high-pitched tone (baby talk).
- Responding: The mother tends to respond verbally to sounds the infant makes.

Initially, the mother may feel herself separate and distant from the child, especially if she does not feel an immediate bond, and the mother should be reassured that these feelings are normal. The following are phases of maternal attachment/bonding:
- Acquaintance - During the acquaintance period (first few days), responding helps the mother to recognize clues the child is giving about needs, such as hunger, and the mother's ability to respond to those needs strengthens the bond and helps the mother gain confidence in her parenting ability. During this time, the infant is also learning to recognize routines, such as breastfeeding when held toward the breast.
- Mutual regulation - During this phase, which may vary in duration, the mother is learning to balance the needs of the infant against her own needs, and she may have some negative feelings, such as resenting her lack of sleep or feeling frustration with the infant's crying. The mother may be afraid to express any negative feelings, fearful that people will think she is a "bad" mother, but these feelings are normal until the mother and infant reach a mutual balance. The ability of the mother and infant to recognize each other's cues and respond to them is termed reciprocity.

Maternal attachment/bonding

Assessment of maternal attachment/bonding should be done prior to discharge so that any issues and interventions can be discussed. In doing the assessment, the nurse evaluates the following:
- Progression in touching and face-to-face in eye contact with extended times and indications of attraction, such as verbally responding to the infant and cuddling the infant. If no progression, then the nurse should assess contributing environmental, cultural, and social factors that may interfere
- Consistency in caring for the infant and seeking both knowledge about and validation of her infant care, adjusting care to the needs of the infant. Sensitivity to infant's needs, such as recognizing discomfort or hunger quickly, and exhibiting pleasure at infant's response to her efforts
- Pleasure in the infant, expressed by calling the infant by name, noting family traits/characteristics, showing overt happiness. If the mother shows displeasure or apathy, this may indicate poor attachment but might also indicate the mother is experiencing pain or weakness

Paternal attachment

Paternal attachment, referred to as engrossment, occurs in many ways similar to maternal attachment. The father may feel pride and wonderment at the child and develop a strong sense of nurturing. Early and frequent contact with the infant promotes engrossment, so the nurse should ensure that the father is not overlooked after delivery but is able to hold, touch, and respond to the child as soon as possible.

Sibling and family attachment

Sibling and family attachment is important. Siblings should be allowed to visit the mother and infant as early as possible and encouraged to hold or care for the infant as appropriate for their ages. Siblings sometimes feel left out or overshadowed by the new infant, so it is important that the parents take time to talk to the siblings and give them attention as well. Grandparents and other family members also form attachment to the infant and should be included.

Parent-infant interaction barriers

There are many barriers to parent-infant interaction, especially with preterm infants or those with genetic disabilities/birth defects that require prolonged hospitalization or treatment. Barriers include:
- Physical separation: When the infant cannot be held or fed, when the child is transported to a different facility outside of the area, or when the mother is discharged and the infant remains hospitalized, this prevents attachment.
- Lack of clear understanding of handicaps/developmental problems: Lack of infant response is sometimes interpreted as rejection, and parents may be frightened by abnormalities.
- Attitude of medical staff: Negative attitudes may cause the parent to grieve rather than attach to the child. Staff members need to encourage the parents to become involved in the child's care and provide stimulation. Staff often needs to demonstrate care to parents, who may be intimidated by the infant's condition and medical needs.
- Environmental overload: The equipment (alarms, ventilators, monitors) and environmental constraints (no chairs) may overwhelm parents.

Values and roles

The following are psychosocial factors affecting family integration:
- Values - Values based on attitudes, ideas, and beliefs often connect family members to common goals. However, these values may be influenced by many external factors, such as education, social norms, and attitudes of peers, other family, and coworkers, so values may change and this may impact family integration.
- Roles - In some families, roles are clearly defined by gender and task (homemaker and breadwinner), but the roles blur or are shared in many families, and in some cases the father becomes the primary caregiver while the mother works. Other common rules include peacemaker, nurturer, and social planner. How these roles are perceived and actualized affects the manner in which a child is integrated into the family.

- Decision making - Family power structures vary widely, but in many families power rests with one person who makes ultimate decisions and whose opinions affect other family members. In many traditional cultures (Hispanic, Asian, Middle Eastern) power lies with the father, a grandparent, or other family member. However, in American society, this may vary because of diversity. Power may be shared or rest with the mother or the father.
- Socioeconomic - Employment trends, marriage rates, and economic trends all affect family integration. Many people have become unemployed and are unable to support their families, resulting in severe stress, which may be exacerbated by the arrival of a new child. The divorce rate is high, leaving many parents with inadequate funds to support a child. Even if both parents are employed, the cost of living continues to escalate, including the cost of caring for a child.

Family types

Types of family include:
- Nuclear - This husband-wife-children model was once the most common family type but is no longer the norm. In this model, the husband is the provider, and the mother stays home to care for the children, but this makes up only about 7% of current American families.
- Dual career/ Dual earner - This model where both parents work is the most common in American society, affecting about 66% of two-parent families. One parent may work more than another or both may work full-time. There may be disparities in income that affect family dynamics.
- Childless - 10% to 15% have no children because of infertility or choice.
- Extended - This may include multigenerational families or shared households with friends, parents, or other relatives. Childcare responsibilities may be shared or primarily assumed by an extended family member, such as a grandparent.
- Extended kin network - Two nuclear families live closely together and share goods and services and support each other, including caring for children. This model is common in the Hispanic community.
- Single parent - This is one of the fastest growing family models. Usually the mother is the single parent, but in some cases it is the father. The single parent may be widowed, divorced, or separated, but more commonly the person has never married. In cases of divorce or abandonment, the child may have minimal or no contact with one parent, often the father. Single parents often face difficulties in trying to support and care for a child and may suffer economic hardship.
- Stepparent - Because of the high rate of divorce, stepparent families are common, and this can result in stress and conflict when a new child enters the picture. There may be jealousy and resentment on the part of siblings and estranged family members. In some cases, families can work together to achieve harmony and provide added support to children.
- Binuclear/ Co-parenting - In this model, children share time between two primarily nuclear families because of joint custody agreements. While this may at times result in conflict, the child benefits from having a continued relationship with both parents.
- Cohabiting - Unmarried heterosexual couples live together. The relationships within this model may vary, with some similar to the nuclear family. In some cases, people are in committed relationships and may avoid marriage because of economic or

personal reasons. A planned child may strengthen the relationship, but an unplanned child may cause conflict.

- Gay/Lesbian - In a few states, gays and lesbians can marry, but in most they cohabit and create families in nontraditional ways. For example, lesbians may use sperm donors. Gay couples often adopt. Children in these families may face social pressures because of their parents' lifestyles, but these children tend to fare as well as those raised in heterosexual households.

Breastfeeding/bottle feeding

Neonates should be fed on demand. Most newborns breastfeed every 2 to 3 hours or bottle feed every 2 to 4 hours (8 to 12 times daily) for 20 to 40 minutes. Over time, the infant will establish a more regular feeding schedule, but this may vary widely.

- Try to recognize clues that the infant is hungry and nurse/feed before the infant begins crying frantically. Signs of hunger include licking, rooting, sucking, making fists, bringing hands to mouth, and bobbing the head.
- Stroke the infant's cheek or lower lip and a hungry infant will usually turn and try to suck the finger.
- Monitor number of diapers per day and stools, as decrease beyond the average normal number may indicate dehydration and inadequate nursing/feeding.
- Observe the infant's behavior closely as some infants nurse for a while and then nap at the breast or take a break before resuming nursing/feeding. A full baby often turns away from the breast/bottle, stops sucking, or resists feeding.

Breastfeeding

Most infants initially breastfeed every 1 to 3 hours but during growth spurts (2 to 3 weeks, 6 weeks, 3 and 6 months) the infant may breastfeed every half to 1 hour for 2 to 3 days, stimulating the breast to increase production. Breastfeeding usually takes 20 to 45 minutes with 15 to 20 minutes on each side. Breastfeeding should begin on the last breast used. Infants may breastfeed more frequently in the late afternoon and evening. Infants should be fed every 3 hours until they regain their birth weight, even if the infant must be awakened. Infants vary in demand schedules. Some eat 5 to 10 times over a 3-hour period and then sleep for about 4 hours. The schedule is less important than ensuring the child breastfeeds 8 to 12 times per 24 hours and appears satisfied. By 8 to 12 weeks, infants begin sleeping longer at night. Some may sleep through the night at 4 months while others continue to breastfeed at night.

Benefits
Breast milk is the food of choice for newborn infants. Colostrum, produced during the first few days after birth, is scant, thick, yellowish, and high in protein and antibody content. Colostrum stimulates the passage of meconium. Transitional milk (days 3 to 14) is thinner and white with a composition closer to mature milk. By the second week, most mothers produce 23 to 27 ounces of bluish-white, mature breast milk. Most neonates nurse every 1 to 3 hours for 20 to 40 minutes. Breast milk provides appropriate amounts of carbohydrate, protein, fat, vitamins, minerals, enzymes, and trace elements. It contains maternal antibodies that help bolster the infant's immature immune system. Breastfed babies have reduced risks of eczema, asthma, obesity, and elevated cholesterol later in life. Breastfeeding enhances the bond between the mother and the infant by physical contact and recognition of communication signals. The maternal cost is an extra 500 calories a day

and extra water. There is no chance of causing kidney damage by mixing formula incorrectly.

Positioning

During breastfeeding, the baby should be turned toward the mother, with the face titled up toward the mother's so they can make eye contact, and the mouth slightly below the nipple, which is pointed toward the baby's upper lip or nostrils. Holds include:
- Cradle: The baby is cradled in the arm on the nursing side with the arm supported by a pillow. The mother uses the opposite hand to guide the nipple and positions the infant toward her.
- Cross-cradle: The hand on the side of the breast used is free to guide the breast while the opposite arm crosses over the baby, and the hand supports the baby's head.
- Football: The infant is tucked under the arm on the nursing side with the arm supporting the baby's back and the hand the head.
- Side-lying: This position is similar to the cradle hold but the mother is reclining on her side, so there is no pressure on the abdomen. Infant is cradled by the arm on the nursing side.

Latching on and let-down
Once the infant is in position, the mother should grasp the breast using a C-hold or U-hold (to make the breast more firm) and lean toward the baby, guiding the nipple toward the infant's mouth. Brushing the nipple against the infant's mouth usually causes the infant to open the mouth and lunge toward the breast. Then, the mother guides the nipple into the infant's mouth while pulling the infant toward the breast. The infant's lower lip should be low on the areola so that the baby latches on to both the areola and the nipple. Suckling stimulates nerves in the areola and nipple, increasing production of prolactin and oxytocin, which in turn stimulate contraction of cells about the areola, causing milk to be ejected in a "let-down" (milk-ejection) reflex (sometimes associated with a tingling sensation), usually within a few minutes of breastfeeding. It may take up to 2 weeks before letdown is efficient.

Neonate's suck swallow sequence
A neonate usually sucks and then swallows when the mouth becomes full. Each suck usually fills the mouth, a suck-to-swallow ratio of 1:1. Infants do not breathe while swallowing, so a 1:1 ratio means the child must breathe quickly, resulting in a rapid suck-hold breath and swallow-breathe sequence. During a swallow, the soft palate raises to block access to the nasal passages, the larynx raises, and the epiglottis covers the airway to prevent aspiration. If milk flow is inadequate, the child may need to suck twice for each swallow (2:1). If the flow is too fast, the child may need to swallow twice or more for each suck (1:2) and some milk may run down the pharynx and into the airway, resulting in aspiration. Additionally, the child may need to swallow so rapidly there is no time to breathe and apnea may occur. A newborn usually sucks twice a second for about a minute and then about one time per second as the milk flow increases.

Feeding cues

The infant gives a number of feeding cues to show hunger. Mothers should be taught to recognize these cues, as it is more difficult for a frantically hungry baby to latch on. Indications include:

- Licking the lips
- Sucking motions of the mouth
- Rooting or bobbing of the head
- Keeping hands in fists
- Bringing hands near mouth or face
- Turning the head toward and trying to suck on a finger stroking the baby's cheek or lower lip.
- Crying (usually the last indication)

Infants who are consistently not receiving adequate nutrition usually appear sleepy and listless. They often stop gaining weight or lose weight. Skin turgor may be poor. Urinary output and stools decrease. The infant may appear disinterested in breastfeeding. On the other hand, an infant that is satisfied usually stops sucking and may turn the head away from the breast or bottle or resist breastfeeding. The infant will appear relaxed and may doze. Some infants take short breaks while feeding/nursing and then resume.

Contraindications

Some maternal contraindications to breastfeeding include:

- Infection with HIV/AIDS
- Use of antiretroviral medications
- Active tuberculosis (not treated)
- Infection with human T-cell lymphotropic virus (II or II)
- Illicit drug use
- Use of chemotherapeutic agents
- Radiation therapy (may require only interruption during treatment)
- Use of other medications that pass into the breast milk and may harm the child.
- Presence of herpes on the breast
- Presence of varicella lesions on the breast (may resume after lesions crust)

Additionally, infants with galactosemia cannot tolerate lactose, which is present in breast milk. Mothers who are ill or become pregnant while breastfeeding should be evaluated on an individual basis to determine if they should continue to breastfeed their infants; mother's with psychiatric disorders, such as schizophrenia or postpartum depression/psychosis, may be unable to breastfeed because of emotional disturbance as well as medications used to treat these conditions.

Complications of breastfeeding

Engorgement: Production of milk sometimes outstrips demand in the first 2 to 3 days as the mother is starting to breastfeed, and the breasts become engorged (enlarged, taut, and painful). The mother should be reassured that this is fairly normal and can be relieved, as new mothers may feel they should stop breastfeeding or be afraid they are doing something wrong. Nursing frequently (every 2 to 3 hours) and gently massaging the breast toward the nipple during breastfeeding should reduce engorgement. If the areola is hard, some milk should be manually expressed to soften the areola before the infant latches on. Breast pumps and heat (except in a shower) may increase engorgement. Cold compresses, acetaminophen, or ibuprofen may provide relief. Engorgement usually recedes within 24 to 48 hours.

Insufficient milk: Only about 1.5% of women are actually physiologically unable to produce sufficient milk for an infant. In almost all cases, the mother is simply not breastfeeding correctly or frequently enough to stimulate milk production.

Blocked milk duct: A palpable localized lump or an area of hard swollen erythematous tissue usually indicates a blocked duct. Causes include breastfeeding the baby in the same position or wearing a constricting or poorly fitting bra. While painful, blocked ducts generally open within 24 to 48 hours with symptoms receding (as opposed to mastitis that tends to worsen). Massaging the affected area while breastfeeding, manually expressing the breast during a warm shower, applying heat to the area, and using a breast pump to completely empty the breast after feeding may all alleviate the blockage. Additionally, while breastfeeding on the affected side, the infant should be positioned so the chin points toward the blocked area (usually using the football position). If blockage is not alleviated, blocked milk ducts may progress to mastitis.

Mastitis: If the breast becomes infected with bacteria, indications include induration, swelling, erythema, increasing fever, and acute pain. Without prompt treatment, painful abscesses may form. The infected area may be localized (sometimes appearing similar to blocked milk duct) or generalized, encompassing the whole breast. The mother may have chills and flu-like symptoms before obvious inflammation of the breast. Usually the mother becomes infected from the infant (most commonly with *Staphylococcus aureus)* so breastfeeding does not endanger the neonate. Treatment includes antibiotics (usually penicillin G, dicloxacillin, or erythromycin) and breastfeeding (or pumping or expressing) on the affected side to prevent abscess formation. Applying heat or massaging the breasts in a warm shower may increase circulation. Pain relief includes alternating warm and cold compresses and acetaminophen or ibuprofen.

Cracked nipples: Nipples often become sore when the mother begins breastfeeding, but this typically reduces in a few days. However, cracked nipples may lead to infection. Causes include:
- Improper latching on of just the nipple and not the areola.
- Use of drying lotions or soaps
- Use of a breast pump with too much suction
- Monilial infection from baby's mouth thrush

Sometimes changing the baby's position or rotating positions during breastfeeding may reduce discomfort. The baby should begin breastfeeding on the least sore nipple as the infant nurses more strongly at first. The breasts should be cleansed only with water and a small amount of breast milk applied to the nipple after nursing unless the baby has thrush. 100% USP modified lanolin (*Lansinoh* or *PureLan*) applied to the nipples may promote healing. It does not need to be removed for breastfeeding. Acetaminophen or ibuprofen may be taken 30 minutes before breastfeeding. Nipple shields should be avoided if possible as they interfere with latching on.

Therapeutic medications while breastfeeding

Virtually all drugs are excreted to some degree (usually 1% to 2% of maternal dose) in the breast milk. Drugs that are highly protein-bound or have molecular weight more than 200 pass less easily into breast milk than lipid-soluble drugs. Breast milk is slightly acidic compared with plasma, so compounds that are weakly alkaline may be present in breast milk in larger amounts than in plasma. Mothers should be advised to take medications after breastfeeding to minimize transfer. Some medications have adverse effects on infants:

- Opiates: Sedation.
- Aspirin: Risk of Reye syndrome.
- Antibiotics: Penicillins may cause diarrhea; tetracyclines, stained/mottled teeth, and chloramphenicol, gray baby syndrome.
- Antifungals: GI symptoms, such as diarrhea, vomiting; blood dyscrasias.
- Cardiovascular drugs: Reserpine may cause diarrhea, bradycardia, lethargy, and respiratory distress; propranolol may cause respiratory depression, bradycardia, or hypoglycemia.
- Psychotherapeutic agents: Sedation, poor feeding. Lithium may cause cyanosis and hypoventilation.
- Ethanol: Lethargy, drowsiness, depressed motor development.
- Stimulants: Irritability and jitteriness. Cocaine may cause neurotoxicity.

Perinatal substance abuse

Mothers who engage in substance abuse should not breastfeed especially under the following circumstances:

- Use large quantities of vasoconstrictive stimulants, such as amphetamines or cocaine
- Drink more than 8 servings of alcohol daily. Binge drinking poses increased risk
- Take sedating opioids (e.g., heroin, benzodiazepine)

Despite concerns, many mothers continue to breastfeed while engaging in substance abuse. In that case, mothers should be educated about their drug of choice and the effects on infants, and on methods to breastfeed as safely as possible. Some safeguards include:

- Encourage mothers to stop injection drug use
- Use drugs only after breastfeeding and use drugs during times the child sleeps longest.
- Express milk during periods of drug use to maintain milk supply
- Pump extra milk during "safe" times to provide feedings to the infant during times of drug use
- Avoid breastfeeding during time the drug is most active. Breastfeeding should be done after the blood level of the drug peaks. For example, alcohol peaks in 30 to 90 minutes. The mother should avoid breastfeeding for 1 to 2 hours for every 2 standard drinks ingested

Infant formulas

A wide variety of infant formulas are available, but the 3 primary types include:
- Cow-milk based formulas (Enfamil, Similac, Good Start): Appropriate for most infants. These are enriched with various components, including vitamins, minerals, iron, tyrosine, phenylalanine, and carnitine
- Soy-based formulas (Isomil, Soyalac, ProSobee, Nursoy): Appropriate for infants with primary lactose deficiency or galactosemia and those allergic to cow-milk based formulas
- Therapeutic formulas (Nutramigen, Pregestimil): Many preparations are available to meet special needs

Formula may be purchased in ready-to-feed bottles or cans that require no preparation, liquid concentrate, or powder. Concentrate and powder require the addition of water, so a clean water supply and ability to measure correctly are necessary to avoid inadequate or unsafe nutrition. Babies who are bottle-fed with formula usually feed less frequently than those who are breastfed. Neonates usually take 2 to 3 ounces of formula ever 3 to 4 hours. Neonates typically require approximately 2.5 ounces of formula for each pound (0.5 kg) of weight within each 24-hour period.

Neonate bottle-feeding

A wide variety of bottle and nipple types is available for bottle-feeding, including some that are shaped to mimic the breast. A mother may try various types to determine which she and the infant prefer. The neonate is usually given the initial feeding when the infant shows signs of hunger. Babies who are formula fed usually awaken every 2 to 5 hours for feedings, but most feed every 3 to 4 hours. Formula is absorbed more slowly than breast milk so the infant may not be hungry as often, but neonates should not go more than 4 hours between feedings because they may become dehydrated. The baby should be fed with the head slightly elevated. The nipple and the area above it must be filled with formula so the baby is not swallowing air. The infant should be burped after every 2 or 3 ounces of formula. Mothers must be cautioned that they should not prop the bottle but should always hold the baby during feedings.

Education for infant care

Choking or gagging
Prevention is important as most choking and gagging episodes can be avoided
- Ensure small hazardous items (pins, cotton balls) or materials (baby powder) are out of reach
- Do NOT prop bottle for feeding
- Burp infant regularly during feedings (breast and bottle)
- Keep baby in upright position with head elevated during feedings
- Check nipple of bottle to ensure it is dripping and not running freely
- If choking, secure infant facedown on forearm, tilted downward, and uses the heel of the hand to thump in the mid back. Repeat as necessary. If choking does not resolve with evidence of breathing immediately, call 9-1-1 and begin CPR

Umbilical cord

The umbilical cord changes color from grayish to brown to black as it dries and finally falls off in about 10 to 14 days:

- Protect the cord from moisture, with top of diaper folded under the cord instead of covering it
- If the cord becomes soiled, wash with mild soap and water, rinse, and dry. (Swabbing with alcohol is still sometimes advised by physicians but is no longer recommended and may increase skin irritation)
- Avoid covering the cord stump with clothing, which may cause irritation
- Give the infant only sponge baths until the cord falls off in about 10 to 14 days
- Report signs of infection, such as erythema, swelling, or purulent discharge

Fontanels

The infant's fontanels (anterior and posterior) are covered by thick membranous tissue and should feel flat but firm:

- Do NOT be afraid to touch the fontanels or cleanse the scalp
- Report bulging above the level of the skull, as this may indicate increased intracranial pressure
- Report a soft fontanel that sinks below the level of the skull, as this may indicate dehydration

Circumcision

Circumcised penis: Circumcision is becoming less common, with only about 50% of male infants now circumcised in the United States. Some people still choose circumcision for religious reasons. Health/hygiene reasons are somewhat controversial. While at one time infants were not thought to experience pain, it is now clear that they do, so circumcision should be done under anesthesia of some type, usually local anesthesia. Typically, the end of the foreskin is swollen and red after circumcision, and some bleeding may persist for 24 hours.

- Change the diaper immediately because urine may cause pain to the open tissue
- Cleanse the area gently with water and pat dry

Noncircumcised penis: The infant's foreskin is different from the adult man's and does not separate and retract until ≥ 5 years old

- Do NOT attempt to retract the foreskin
- Do NOT use cotton swabs to clean
- Wash the penis with soap and water or just water during the routine bath

Burping

Both breastfed and bottle-fed babies require burping because they swallow air when feeding, although bottle fed babies tend to require more burping. Infants often show indications (grimacing, squirming, spitting up, and crying) that they are uncomfortable and need to burp

- Burp the infant routinely after 2 or 3 ounces of formula or after breastfeeding on one breast
- Position the infant on the shoulder (with a burp cloth under the infant's head) and gently pat or rub the infant's back

- Change to a different position if the baby does not burp (opposite shoulder or with the infant sitting on the lap and supported by one hand while the other hand pats or rubs the infant's back)

Positioning

Infants should be placed on their backs for sleeping. Sleeping on the stomach increases risk of sudden infant death syndrome (SIDS):
- Position the infant on the back when unattended or sleeping, but alternate the direction the head faces to prevent one side of the head from flattening (positional molding).
- Provide supervised time each day with the infant lying on the abdomen (only on firm surfaces) to strengthen head and neck muscles and to prevent positional molding.
- Hold the infant rather than leaving in carriers.
- Position baby in side-lying position (alternating from one side to the other), using specially designed supports to maintain the position.

Infant car seat

All infants, regardless of age, must be placed properly in an infant car seat during transit. Holding an infant while the car is in motion is not safe. Car seats should be new or in very good condition and fastened according to manufacturer's guidelines to ensure safety.
- Place the car seat in the back seat and away from any side airbags
- Always securely buckle the child into the seat
- Face the infant seat toward the rear of the car
- Recline the seat so that the infant's head does not fall forward
- Place padding around (not under) the infant if the infant slouches to one side
- Place blankets OVER the straps and buckles, not under

Bath

The infant should receive sponge baths until the cord falls off (10 to 14 days) and then a bath in an infant tub (NOT in an adult tub). Mild soap/shampoo intended for babies or just water alone may be used for the bath.
- Make sure the environmental temperature is warm
- Fill tub with 2 to 3 inches of water
- ALWAYS check water temperature to make sure it is warm and NOT hot
- Set hot water heaters $\leq 120°$ F to prevent inadvertent scalding
- Support the baby during the bath with one arm under upper back to support the neck and head while holding the infant under the axilla
- Pour water over the child with the free hand and use that hand to wash the hair and the body.
- Lift the baby from the tub and wrap in a towel to dry
- Dry thoroughly, making sure all skin folds and crevices are dry to prevent irritation and rashes
- Avoid use of lotions or creams

Fecal elimination

The first stool (meconium) is usually passed within 48 hours and is black and tarry-looking. The stool then transitions to greenish as the baby breastfeeds or takes formula, and by the third day the stool is usually yellow or yellow-green for breastfed babies and yellow or light brown for formula-fed babies. Typically, babies have 2 to 3 stools daily by day 3 and ≥ 4 daily by day 5, but this may vary.

- Report abnormalities, such as bloody stools, watery stools, very hard stool, clay-colored or whitish stools, black stools (after meconium has passed), and "currant jelly" stools
- Cleanse skin thoroughly after defecation with mild soap and water, plain water, or unscented baby wipes
- Examine skin carefully for irritation

Diaper rash

Diaper rash usually results from leaving the infant in soiled/wet diapers and/or not adequately cleansing the skin, although breastfed infants sometimes react to foods the mother has eaten. A rash may also indicate an allergic response to baby wipes or other products, such as lotions or creams. Antibiotics may cause diaper rash. In some cases, a fungal infection may occur, usually characterized by red, weepy open areas. Purulent discharge may indicate infection.

- Change diapers as soon as possible when wet or soiled
- Cleanse skin gently with water
- Remove diaper and expose skin to air whenever possible
- Apply barrier cream or ointment especially formulated for diaper rash to prevent or treat diaper rash
- Contact physician if rash worsens and does not respond to treatment as antifungals, cortisone, or topical antibiotics may be indicated

Urinary elimination and cradle cap

Elimination (urinary): Urination is estimated according to the number of wet diapers in a 24-hour period. Typically, the infant has 1 wet diaper the first day, 2 the next, and so on until urination stabilizes at 6 to 8 wet diapers by about day 6.

- Check diaper frequently. Infants often urinate during or after feeding
- Change diapers when wet, gently cleansing skin with mild soap and water, plain water, or unscented baby wipes

Cradle cap: Cradle cap may appear as scaly, crusted, or flaky skin on the scalp and other parts of the face. It is not contagious and usually clears by 1 or 2 months. It is not usually a sign of poor hygiene.

- Cleanse scalp or affected areas thoroughly, gently rubbing the area with a terry cloth or brushing to loosen crust or flakes
- If persistent, try softening the crusts with olive oil, leave for 15 minutes, and then brush or gently comb to loosen crusts or flakes. Finally, wash with baby shampoo.

Nonnutritive sucking

Nonnutritive sucking occurs when an infant sucks on an item such as a pacifier or his/her own fist. Nonnutritive sucking is not associated with nutritional intake, but it is an important method of self-quieting and begins in the uterus at about 29 weeks of gestation. Extremely premature infants often lack basic neurodevelopmental capabilities, and cannot coordinate sucking, swallowing, and breathing simultaneously. Typically, the ability to suck and swallow in a coordinated fashion is not present until 32 to 34 weeks of gestation. Premature infants should be encouraged to perform nonnutritive sucking during the gavage feeding process if they can accomplish it. Benefits of nonnutritive sucking include:

- Improved digestion of enteral feeds because digestive enzyme release is stimulated
- Facilitated development of coordinated nutritive sucking behavior
- Calming of the distressed infant

Safe positioning

Infants should be placed on their backs for sleeping. Sleeping on the stomach increases risk of sudden infant death syndrome (SIDS).

- Position the infant on the back when unattended or sleeping, but alternate the direction the head faces to prevent one side of the head from flattening (positional molding)
- Provide supervised time each day with the infant lying on the abdomen (only on firm surfaces) to strengthen head and neck muscles and to prevent positional molding
- Hold the infant rather than leaving in carriers
- Position baby in side-lying position (alternating from one side to the other), using specially designed supports to maintain the position

Special needs infant

Family involvement and education are vital for successful discharge of the special needs infant to ensure proper care. Bringing home a premature infant or one who has special needs is a daunting task for any parent. Before discharge, the following should be done:

- Educate the parents or guardian about appropriate caring methods
- Explain how to interpret the infant's cues concerning his needs and how to respond appropriately
- Point out the different states of alertness during their infant's sleep and wake cycles. Identify the appropriate times and methods for infant interaction
- Coach the parents to ensure they perform each skill correctly and retain it. Observe interaction between the infant and parents in the nursery to help ensure continued wellness of the infant after discharge
- Encourage kangaroo care immediately after birth for stable newborns because it is an excellent method to foster bonding between the neonate and the mother. For neonates who require resuscitation and medical intervention, delay kangaroo care until the neonate is stable
- If the parents are not ready, contact social services for follow-up

Oral contraceptives

There are many methods of birth control, including the use of condoms, intrauterine devices, spermicides, and barriers, such as diaphragms, sponges, and cervical caps, but hormonal contraceptives are commonly used. There are 2 types of oral contraceptives, but there are many different brands with differing amounts of hormones:

- Combined (estrogen [ethinyl estradiol] and progestin): These may be monophasic (constant doses), biphasic (constant estrogen but increase of progestin on day 10), or triphasic (varying doses of both)
- Progestin only: These have fewer side effects than combined forms, but can increase estrogen levels and incidence of thrombosis

Oral contraceptives are contraindicated for those who smoke or have evidence or history of breast cancer, coronary artery disease, or elevated cholesterol because they are associated with increased risk of thrombosis. Common side effects (depending upon the particular drug) include an increase in acne and facial hair growth, weight increase, rash or itching, amenorrhea, decrease in libido, headache, nausea, and breakthrough bleeding. Changing to a different contraceptive may alleviate symptoms.

Contraception

Newer methods of contraception include injectable, ring, and patch contraceptives. One primary advantage is that the woman does not need to remember to take pills, but risks are similar to oral contraceptives:

- NuvaRing is a vaginal ring that is inserted vaginally and left in place over the cervix for 3 weeks. It is removed for the 4th week, during which there may be withdrawal bleeding. It is as effective as oral contraceptives.
- OrthoEvra is a small adhesive patch that is applied to the torso, chest (excluding the breasts), arms, or thighs every week for 3 weeks and then the 4th week is patch free. It is as effective as oral contraceptives.
- Depo-Provera is injectable medroxyprogesterone acetate that is given every 13 weeks. It is contraindicated with a history of deep vein thrombosis or smoking. It may relieve symptoms of endometriosis.

Emergency contraception

Females who have had unprotected sexual intercourse, consensual or rape, are at risk for pregnancy and may desire emergency contraception. Emergency contraception inhibits ovulation and prevents pregnancy rather than aborting a pregnancy. Emergency contraceptives have been marketed for use 72 hours or less but recent studies indicate they are effective for 120 hours or less. Options include:

- Plan B or Next Choice (Levonorgestrel) - The first pill (0.75 mg) must be taken ≤ 72 hours (3 days) after unprotected intercourse and the second (also 0.75 mg) 12 hours later or both pills may be taken in the same initial dose.
- Plan B One-Step (Levonorgestrel) - One pill (1.5 mg) only is taken ≤ 72 hours (3 days) after unprotected intercourse. This is now used more commonly than Plan B.
- EllaOne (Ulipristal acetate) - One pill (30 mg) is taken ≤ 120 hours (5 days) after unprotected intercourse.

A follow-up pregnancy test should be done if the person does not menstruate within 3 weeks because the failure rate is about 1.5%. Adverse effects include nausea (relieved by taking medication with meals or with an antiemetic), breast tenderness, and irregular bleeding.

Condoms and IUDs

Male and female condom: These are more effective if used with spermicide, but nonoxynol-9 (N-9) should be avoided because it interferes with protection against sexually transmitted diseases. Patients should have instruction in proper use to avoid semen leaking from the male condom. Condoms are 80% to 90% effective.

Intrauterine device (IUD): IUDs are usually T-shaped and are inserted through the cervix into the uterus (with the attached string palpable at the cervical opening). IUDs prevent pregnancy by causing a local inflammatory response that prevents fertilization. Some are plastic, but ParaGard is copper, which has antisperm effects and can be left in place for up to 10 years. Mirena releases levonorgestrel (synthetic progestin) and can be left in place for 5 years. It can be used in smokers, but there may be some adverse effects because of the hormone: acne, increased facial hair, and thickening of cervical mucosa. IUDs are 95% to 99% effective. Adverse effects of IUDs include abnormal bleeding, discharge, or infection.

Diaphragm

This round device has a flexible supporting ring and a dome-like latex cup (requiring latex allergy assessment). The concave surface (facing the cervix) is coated with spermicide before the diaphragm is inserted. The diaphragm is fitted to the individual using sized fitting rings during a pelvic exam so it seats properly below cervix and is held in place by vaginal muscles. Diaphragms range in size from 50 to 90 mm. They should not be placed more than 2 hours prior to intercourse because spermicide loses effectiveness. Diaphragms are left in place for at least 6 hours after intercourse (but not more than 12 hours). Each act of intercourse requires additional insertion of spermicide vaginally. The diaphragm should be washed with soap and water after use and inspected under bright light for tears or holes prior to each use. The diaphragm is 85% to 95% effective if used properly. Changes in weight or pregnancy can alter size requirements, so diaphragms should be refitted when either of these has occurred.

Contraceptive devices

Cervical cap
This latex cap is smaller than the diaphragm (22 to 35 mm) and more cone-shaped, and it fits over the cervix rather than below it. Like the diaphragm, it is used with spermicide. It may cause cervical irritation, so women may need Pap tests more frequently (every 3 months). It has the advantage of being able to stay in place for up to 48 hours, but leaving it in for long periods increases the risk of vaginitis and toxic shock syndrome. Cervical caps do not require additional spermicide for each act of intercourse and are 85% 95% effective.

Contraceptive sponge
This is a donut-shaped spongy barrier device that contains nonoxynol-9 (N-9), so it is 85% to 95% effective but does not protect against STDs. The sponge has a concave central

indentation on one side that fits over the cervix to act as a barrier. The outside has a string for easy removal. The sponge is left in place for 6 hours after intercourse but not >30 hours.

Contraceptive practices

Coitus interruptus
This requires withdrawing the penis from the vagina prior to ejaculation. It is a frequently used method of birth control, especially among teenagers, but it is completely unreliable as sperm may leak prior to ejaculation.

Rhythm methods
Using rhythm methods requires determining when the woman ovulates and abstinence from sex during the fertile phase. Pregnancy rates are about 40% so this method is only advised if couples are very disciplined, monitor their cycles carefully, and are willing to abstain from sex for long periods during each cycle. This method is often used because of religious restrictions against artificial birth control. Ovulation detection kits are available OTC. They detect the enzyme guaiacol peroxidase in cervical mucosa. This indicates ovulation will occur in about 6 days. These kits, however, are more reliable for those attempting to become pregnant than to avoid pregnancy.

Sterilization

Vasectomy
The male's vas deferens are clipped or severed and then tied or sealed under local anesthetic. The procedure is done with one central puncture or bilateral incisions. Other birth control methods must be used for 4 to 6 weeks. It may take up to 36 ejaculations to clear remaining sperm. A sperm count is done at 6 weeks with follow-up at 6 and 12 months to check for recanalization that might restore fertility. Discomfort is usually minimal. Complications include infection, pain, hematoma, and recurrent epididymitis. Reversal techniques are 30% to 85% effective.

Tubal ligation
Tubal ligation seals the fallopian tubes to prevent conception. Various methods are available, including clipping, silicone rings, cauterization, and surgical cutting and realigning. Tubal ligation is often done during cesarean delivery or shortly after vaginal birth because the tubes are easier to isolate after pregnancy. Complications include infection, pain, perforated or burned bowel, and hemorrhage. Reversal techniques are 45% to 80% effective.

Postpartal voiding problems

Voiding problems, such as bladder retention or inability to initiate urine flow or completely empty the bladder, are common after delivery because of periurethral edema. Dysuria is usually transitory. Mothers should be encouraged to try to urinate within the first hour after delivery. The mother should empty the bladder at least every 4 to 6 hours, and the bladder should not be palpable. Pouring warm water over the perineum or a warm shower may help relax muscles enough to promote urination. The time and amount of voiding should be recorded. Normal volume for each urination is 300 to 400 mL. Smaller amounts may indicate dehydration or incomplete bladder emptying, which may be verified by ultrasound. Repeated catheterization more than 2 times in 24 hours should be avoided. If the mother is still unable to urinate after straight catheterizations, then an indwelling catheter along with prophylactic administration of ampicillin may be considered.

Postpartal hemorrhage

Postpartal hemorrhage may be early (24 hours or less) or late (6 weeks or less). Normal blood loss with vaginal delivery is about 500 mL and with cesarean about 1000 mL. Blood loss is difficult to estimate because it is mixed with amniotic fluid and mucus, and hemorrhage may be internal and not obvious on examination. Usual indications of hemorrhage, such as increased pulse, decreased blood pressure, and decreased output of urine, may be delayed until about 2 L of blood loss. A significant drop in hematocrit (10 points) is indicative of hemorrhage. Early hemorrhage poses more risk of mortality than late hemorrhage. When hemorrhage is suspected, such as with steady flow of lochia rubra, the woman's vital signs should be checked every 5 to 15 minutes and perineal pads weighed (1 mL of blood weighs about 1 g). A soft boggy uterus should be massaged frequently to maintain firmness, with clots expressed. IV access should be maintained. Urinary output less than 30 mL/h should be reported to the physician.

Causes of postpartal hemorrhage are as follows:
- Early:
  - Uterine atony: Most common with multiple gestations, prolonged labor, labor induction, anesthesia, preeclampsia, and placenta previa. Uterine contractions are necessary to occlude blood flow to placenta.
  - Genital lacerations: Lacerations may be undetected, or the episiotomy may continue to slowly ooze blood.
  - Hematomas: Trauma to blood vessels may occur, especially with pudendal anesthesia, forceps or vacuum-assisted delivery, macrosomia, and prolonged second stage of labor.
  - Inversion of uterus: This is rare but may occur with weak uterine muscles, extended labor, anesthesia, magnesium sulfate, and manual removal of placenta with excess traction. Rupture of uterus: This is also rare but can occur with previous cesarean delivery, multiparity, and induction (oxytocin). Abnormal implantation of placenta.
  - Coagulopathies: DIC may occur in response to blood loss or cause blood loss.
- Late:
  - Subinvolution of placental implantation site (failure of implantation site to shrink and heal): Leaves open tissue that may bleed.
  - Retained placental tissue: Bleeding occurs when it sloughs from implantation site.

Postpartal hematoma

A hematoma may form in the perineal area after delivery, especially if an episiotomy is present. Hematomas may form anywhere from the vulva to the upper vagina because of trauma. Severe vulvar or vaginal pain that is not relieved by usual analgesia may indicate a hematoma is forming. Hematomas must be monitored carefully. Those less than 5 cm may resolve over time. Ice packs may help to reduce discomfort. Vital signs should be monitored carefully for signs of hemorrhage. Larger hematomas require surgical excision of the most dependent portion and drainage. The incision may be closed or left open with drains or packing to prevent recurrent hematoma. If the hematoma is at the site of the episiotomy, then the suture line must be opened to identify the site of bleeding.

Postpartal infections

Endometritis (Endometrial inflammation) may result from cesarean delivery, PROM, repeated vaginal examination, fetal scalp electrode, instruments (forceps or vacuum), high-risk status of mother (drug use, smoker, poor nutrition), or preexisting vaginal infection. Indications include foul-smelling or scant lochia (depending on organism), uterine tenderness, temperature elevations (sawtooth pattern) 38.3° to 40°C, tachycardia, and chills. Parametritis (Pelvic cellulitis/Peritonitis) is an infection of connective tissue of broad ligament or all pelvic structures that may result from bacterial invasion of cervical laceration or pelvic vein thrombophlebitis. Abscess may form. Indications include chills high fever (38.9° to 40°C), abdominal pain, uterine subinvolution, local and rebound tenderness, tachycardia, abdominal distention, nausea and vomiting. Urinary infections may result from birth trauma, urinary retention, and contamination (catheter). Indications include dysuria, fever, and urinary retention. Wound infections may result from contamination of lacerations, episiotomy, and cesarean delivery incisions. Indications include erythema, local pain, purulent discharge, edema, and (rare) dehiscence

Postpartal thrombophlebitis

Thrombophlebitis may occur in the postpartal period with indications of septic thrombophlebitis typically evident 3 to 7 days after delivery. Clot formation occurs in the vessel walls, leading to occlusion and inflammation. Fibrinolytic activity decreases during pregnancy to prevent hemorrhage occurring with delivery; however, this change can promote development of deep vein thrombosis and thrombophlebitis. Additionally, inactivity and bed rest increase risk. Coagulation usually returns to normal within about 3 days after delivery, so later onset often relates to other factors, such as a history of varicose veins. Superficial thrombophlebitis is usually evident by observable symptoms and poses less risk of clots breaking free and migrating than deep vein thrombophlebitis.

Indications include:
- Femoral: Localized pain and swelling with edema of the leg from impaired circulation, often accompanied by fever and chills
- Pelvic: Abdominal pain, fever, and chills, as well as generalized lethargy and malaise

Treatment varies depending on size and type but may include heat, anticoagulation, compression (stockings), elevation of affected limb, and limitations on activities.

Psychosocial impact of fetal/neonatal problems

Siblings should be included and parents encouraged to bring them to visit and interact, as much as possible, with the neonate. If the neonate has abnormalities, this may cause stress to the siblings. Younger children may be hostile and older children ashamed. Children may feel guilty about their responses, and they may feel neglected as parents go through the stages of grief and are unable to provide the support that the siblings need. In some cases, parents may express their concern by focusing their anxiety on one of the siblings, becoming hypercritical. In these cases, staff may need to intervene by discussing observations with the parents and encouraging other family members to provide support to the siblings. Parents' groups that involve the entire family can be very helpful. Whenever possible, children should be included in education and demonstrations and encouraged to ask questions. Age-appropriate books and other materials that explain medical conditions and treatments should be available for siblings.

Steps to decrease family stress

Having a neonate admitted to the neonatal intensive care unit is a very stressful event for a family because it interrupts family interactions and the bonding process that occur when a neonate goes home to spend time with family members. Steps to decrease family stress and encourage bonding between the neonate, mother, and family include:

- Have facilities available for families to stay close to their infant to encourage bonding
- Maintain a play area for siblings so they are not isolated from parents
- Encourage breastfeeding or pumping if possible
- Permit liberal visiting times for family members
- If it is known before birth that the infant will require critical care, let the family visit the unit and ask questions
- Give the family contact information for support groups comprised of other parents who have children with similar illnesses
- Encourage hands-on parental care, including kangaroo care, by both parents

Kübler-Ross' Five Stages of Grief

Grief is a normal response to the death or severe illness/abnormality of an infant or fetus. How a person deals with grief is very personal, and each person will grieve differently. Elisabeth Kübler-Ross identified five stages of grief in *On Death and Dying* (1969). A person may not go through each stage but usually goes through two of the five stages:

- Denial - The parents may be resistant to information and unable to accept that an infant is dying/impaired or believe that the infant is not theirs. They may act stunned, immobile, or detached and may be unable to respond appropriately or remember what is said, often repeatedly asking the same questions.
- Anger - As reality becomes clear, parents may react with pronounced anger, directed inward or outward. Women, especially, may blame themselves and self-anger may lead to severe depression and guilt; they assume blame because of some action before or during pregnancy. Outward anger, more common in men, may be expressed as overt hostility.
- Bargaining - This involves if-then thinking (often directed at a deity): "If I go to church every day, then God will prevent this." Parents may change doctors, trying to change the outcome.
- Depression - As the parents begin to accept the loss, they may become depressed, feeling no one understands, and overwhelmed with sadness. They may be tearful or crying and may withdraw or ask to be left alone.
- Acceptance - This final stage represents a form of resolution and often occurs outside of the medical environment after months. Parents are able to resume their normal activities and lose the constant preoccupation with their infant. They are able to think of the infant without severe pain. With a disabled infant, acceptance may be delayed because of daily challenges and reminders.

Methods to support parents/family

Parents/families of dying infants often do not receive adequate support from nursing staff, who feel unprepared for dealing with parental/familial grief and unsure of how provide comfort, but parents/families are in desperate need of this support:
- Before death:
  - Stay with the family and sit quietly, allowing them to talk, cry, or interact if they desire
  - Avoid platitudes: "His suffering will be over soon"
  - Avoid judgmental reactions to what family members say or do and realize that anger, fear, guilt, and irrational behavior are normal responses to acute grief and stress
  - Show caring by touching the infant and encouraging family to do the same
  - Note: Touching hands, arms, or shoulders of family members can provide comfort, but follow clues of the family
  - Provide referrals to support groups if available
- Time of death:
  - Reassure family that all measures have been taken to ensure the infant's comfort.
  - Express personal feeling of loss, "She was such a sweet baby, and I'll miss her" and allow family to express feelings and memories.
  - Provide information about what is happening during the dying process, explaining death rales, Cheyne-Stokes respirations, etc.
  - Alert family members to imminent death if they are not present. Assist to contact clergy/spiritual advisors.
  - Respect feelings and needs of parents, siblings, and other family.
- After death:
  - Encourage parents/family members to stay with the infant as long as they wish to hold the infant and/or say goodbye. Use the infant's name when talking to the family. Assist them to make arrangements, such as contacting a funeral home.
  - If an autopsy is required, discuss with the family and explain when it will take place.
  - If organ donation is to occur, assist the family to make arrangements. Encourage family members to grieve and express emotions. Send card or condolence note.

Grief

<u>Types</u>
Grief can anticipatory, incongruent, or delayed:
- Anticipatory grief: occurs when a child is diagnosed with a terminal illness. The parent begins to mourn over the loss of the child before he or she dies.
- Incongruent grief: occurs when the mother and the father are "out of synch" in their grieving process, stressing their relationship. It may be due to the differences in how men and women grieve, or it may be because the woman typically bonds with the infant during the pregnancy, while the father bonds after the child is born.

- Delayed grief: occurs when the grieving process is postponed months to years after the loss of a child. Initially, the parent may not be able to grieve appropriately, because of an inability to cope, or the pressing need to care for other family members.

Gender differences
When faced with the death of a child, men and women generally grieve differently:
- Women are often more expressive about their loss and more emotional. They are more likely to look for support from others. Men often grieve in a more solitary and cognitive manner. They are generally more oriented to fact gathering or problem solving.
- The bond that develops between a pregnant woman and the fetus is unique and generally very intense. The father often forms a stronger bond after the birth of the child.

When one parent does not grieve in the same fashion as the other (incongruent grieving) this may be a source of conflict in their marriage. How a person acts on the outside is not always a true indicator of how a person is feeling on the inside.

<u>Grieving family factors</u>
The emotions that individuals and families experience with the loss or severe illness/disability of an infant are varied and dependent on many factors that influence grief:
- Cultural influences: Different cultures have their own practices and beliefs concerning sickness, death, and dying, and varying rituals and ceremonies for processing loss.
- Family system: The family's composition, the roles of various members, and economic circumstances affect its expression of grief. A large family with extended community support processes grief differently than a single mother living far from home.
- Siblings: The impact on other children in the family must be considered rather than concentrating on the parents alone.
- History of loss: Many diseases have a genetic component, and this may not be the first child to be affected

Postpartum depression

Postpartum major mood disorder, commonly referred to as postpartum depression, occurs in more than 10% of mothers. Onset may occur any time within the first year, but is most common around week 4 postpartum, before the onset of menses. Duration varies but is usually 3 to 14 months (half symptomatic at 6 months). Risk factors include primiparity, history of depression, bipolar disease, or previous postpartum depression, lack of stable and supportive social and family relationships, family history of psychiatric illness, and ambivalence about pregnancy. Symptoms are typical of depression and include sadness, crying, insomnia or excess sleeping, difficulty concentrating or making decisions, phobias, anxiety, lack of interest in activities, and feeling out of control or helpless. The mother may be irritable and hostile, especially toward the child. She may also be suicidal. Treatment may include psychotherapy, antidepressants, antipsychotics, and/or lithium. In some cases, the child may need to be cared for by others until the mother's depression lessens.

Postpartum psychosis

Postpartum psychosis may occur up to 3 months postpartum but symptoms are usually evident within the first 3 weeks with sudden onset of psychotic symptoms, such as delusions, hallucinations, insomnia, anorexia, paranoia, and suicidal and/or homicidal ideation. Postpartum psychosis is a medical emergency that often requires hospitalization; in 4% of cases, mothers have committed infanticide, sometimes because of voices urging them to do so. The mother should be carefully supervised when caring for their children until symptoms have abated, or the children should be removed from the mother until the mother stabilizes. While postpartum psychosis is most common in mothers with a history of mental illness (such as schizophrenia or bipolar disease), it can occur in mothers with no such history. The cause is unclear but may be a combination of hormonal imbalance and stress/anxiety. Treatment includes psychotherapy, mood stabilizers, antipsychotics, and benzodiazepines. Antidepressants may cause mood cycling if psychosis is associated with bipolar disorder.

Postpartal complications

While health factors are of primary importance during pregnancy, sociocultural variables, including poverty, inadequate nutrition, inadequate prenatal care, and cultural beliefs regarding pregnancy may increase risk in the antepartal, intrapartal, and postpartal period, so these must also be assessed. The following are postpartal high-risk factors:

- Preeclampsia - Preeclampsia results in hypertension, increased central nervous irritability and the need for bed rest after delivery, increasing the risk of thrombophlebitis.
- Diabetes mellitus - Insulin regulation must be monitored carefully because the mother may experience periods of hypoglycemia or hyperglycemia. Diabetes is also associated with decreased or slower healing.
- Cardio-vascular disorders - Complications may vary, depending on the type of disorder, but increased maternal exhaustion and the need for increased rest are common.
- Cesarean delivery - The mother needs increased protein to promote healing. She may experience increased pain, which may limit activity, increasing risk of thrombophlebitis. The invasive procedure increases risk of infection and usually prolongs hospital stay.
- Uterine overdistention - Uterine overdistention most often relates to multiple gestations or hydramnios. The mother has increased risk of hemorrhage and anemia, as well as increased stretching and damage to abdominal muscles and increased intensity of afterpains.
- Abruptio placentae and placenta previa - Both conditions are associated with increased risk of hemorrhage and anemia, with decreased uterine contractions after birth and increased risk of infection.
- Precipitous labor (< 3 hours) - Because dilatation may be inadequate, there is increased risk of laceration and hemorrhage.
- Prolonged labor (> 24) - The mother may experience exhaustion and inability to push. Risk of infection and nutritional and fluid depletion increase. Pressure may result in increased bladder atony and/or associated trauma.
- Difficult birth - The mother may experience exhaustion and increased risk of laceration, hematoma, hemorrhage, and anemia.

- Placental retention - Retention of the placenta increases risk of hemorrhage and infection.
- Prolonged lithotomy position - Lying too long with legs elevated in stirrups increases risk of thrombophlebitis.

Cesarean delivery care

The mother who has had a cesarean birth has both routine postpartal and surgical needs. The mother should deep breathe and cough (while supporting the abdomen with a pillow) and use an incentive spirometer every 2 to 4 hours during the daytime for the first few days. The mother should sit on the side of the bed within 12 hours of surgery and ambulate within 24 hours. Pain management with patient-controlled analgesia, oral and parenteral medications, and/or relaxation techniques help the mother to ambulate and care for her infant. Epidural analgesia may continue for 24 hours after delivery and must be monitored carefully. Flatus and abdominal distention are common complaints, so the mother should avoid carbonated beverages and drinking through straws. Taking an antiflatulent (*Mylicon*), turning frequently, rocking, or lying on the left side may help to expel gas. The mother should be encouraged to breastfeed but may be more comfortable sitting with the baby supported by a pillow or side lying to prevent pressure on the incision.

Diabetes mellitus

Mothers with diabetes mellitus require careful evaluation but should be encouraged to be as independent as possible in monitoring their own blood sugars and taking medications, such as insulin. Insulin requirements usually drop by 50% to 75% in the 24 hours after delivery because of the drop in hormone levels, so monitoring glucose levels and adjusting insulin dosage are important to prevent insulin reactions. The insulin needs should be reestablished over the next few days, taking into consideration diet and exercise. Diabetic mothers should be encouraged to breastfeed. Insulin needs while breastfeeding are often decreased even with increased caloric intake, so home glucose monitoring and adjustment of insulin doses must continue after discharge. With gestational diabetes, insulin can usually be discontinued after childbirth with glucose levels monitored and oral medications tried if necessary, although oral antihyperglycemics are contraindicated with breastfeeding.

Cardiac disease

Labor may be very taxing for the woman with cardiac disease, and she is often exhausted after birth. The postpartal period can place the mother at increased risk of complications because the changes in uterine and venous pressure increase both cardiac output and blood volume, and this can lead to decompensation within 48 hours after delivery. Vital signs must be monitored frequently and the patient positioned with the head elevated in the semi-Fowler or side-lying position. Unless precluded by medications, the mother should be encouraged to breastfeed, but the nurse may need to provide extra assistance in positioning and burping the infant to help the mother conserve energy. Adequate fluids, dietary fiber, and stool softeners prevent constipation and straining. The mother should be educated about heart disease and postpartal complications, such as hemorrhage or thrombophlebitis, which may increase the risk of heart failure.

HIV/AIDS

Mothers infected with HIV/AIDS and asymptomatic prior to pregnancy usually have no added risk for acceleration of their disease, but increased risk occurs if the CD4 count was already low. Because about half of neonatal infections occur during birth and delivery, the HIV/AIDS mother may have an elective cesarean delivery at 38 weeks. Routine care should be provided, always using standard precautions. The mother is at increased postpartal risk of hemorrhage, urinary and endometrial/pelvic infections, and poor wound healing, and requires careful evaluation for complications. The mother should be educated about all aspects of her disease and the implications and need for follow-up care for both her and her infant. Mothers should be advised not to breastfeed; the virus may be transmitted through breast milk. Prior to discharge the mother should receive referrals to social services that can provide support.

CDC 2007 Guideline for Isolation Precautions (standard precautions)
The CDC 2007 Guideline for Isolation Precautions includes both standard precautions that apply to all patients and transmission-based precautions for those with known or suspected infections, such as HIV/AIDS. Standard precautions should be utilized during treatment for all patients because all body fluids (sweat, urine, feces, blood, sputum) and nonintact skin and mucous membranes may be infected:
- Hand hygiene - Wash hands before and after each patient contact.
- Protective equipment - Use personal protective equipment (PPE), such as gloves, gowns, and masks, eye protection, and/or face shields, depending on the patient's condition and degree of exposure.
- Respiratory hygiene/cough etiquette - Educate staff, patients, family, and visitors.
- Post instructions (language appropriate). Utilize source control measures, such as covering cough, disposing of tissues, using surgical mask on person coughing or on staff to prevent inhalation of droplets, and properly disposing of dressings and used equipment. Wash hands after contacting respiratory secretions. Maintain a distance of > 3 feet from coughing person when possible.
- Safe injection practice - Use sterile single-use needle and syringe one time only and discard safely.

The Neonate

The Normal Newborn

Modified Ballard score overview

The modified Ballard score is used to estimate maturity and gestational age in newborns. It is most reliable when performed within the first 12 hours of life. The Ballard score was modified to include evaluation of extremely premature infants with gestational ages as low as 20 weeks (score -10) and as high as 50 weeks (score 44). It scores 6 measurements of neuromuscular maturity and 6 signs of physical maturity on a scale of -1 to 4 or 5 (depending upon the category).

The total score indicates the estimated gestational age for that infant:
- Neuromuscular measurements:
  - Supine posture
  - Square window (wrist)
  - Arm recoil
  - Popliteal angle
  - Scarf sign
  - Heel to ear
- Physical signs of maturity:
  - Skin characteristics
  - Presence or absence of lanugo
  - Appearance of plantar feet surfaces
  - Presence or absence of breast buds
  - Eye and ear characteristics
  - Genitalia (male and female) characteristics

The six neuromuscular measurements are as follows:
- 1 - Observation of the infant's posture while lying supine indicates the total amount of muscle tone the infant possesses. Increased amounts of flexion of the elbows and knees correlates with increased gestational age.
- 2 - Square window test measures the resistance to stretching of extensor muscles in the infant's forearm. Increased ability for the tester to flex the infant's wrist correlates with greater gestational age.
- 3 - Arm recoil test measures the tone of the biceps muscles. Increased amount of arm recoil (flexion by the infant after the infant's arms are extended) correlates with greater gestational age.
- 4 - Popliteal angle measurement assesses the flexor tone of the knee joint. Increased resistance to flexion at the knee is associated with greater gestational age.
- 5 - Scarf sign test measures the tone of shoulder flexor muscles. Increased resistance to movement of the infant's arm across the chest is associated with greater gestational age.
- 6 - Heel to ear test measures the tone of pelvic girdle muscles. Increased resistance to movement of the infant's foot to the ear is associated with greater gestational age.

The six physical signs of maturity are as follows:

- 1 - Skin: Immature infants have thin, transparent skin. The vernix caseosa begins development at the beginning of the third trimester. Dried, cracked skin occurs as this protective coating disappears after the 40th week.
- 2 - Lanugo: Fine, usually unpigmented hairs begin to appear at 24 to 25 weeks of gestation and thin as the neonate matures.
- 3 - Plantar surface of feet. Very immature infants have no creases on the soles of their feet. Creases develop first on the anterior portion and more mature infants will have creases over the entire sole.
- 4 - Breast buds: Fatty tissue underneath the areola that increases in size as the fetus matures.
- 5 - Ears: Increased cartilage content produces a more rigid pinna; ear recoil increases as the infant matures.
- 6:
  - Male genitalia: The testes descend from the abdomen into the scrotum at 30 weeks of gestation and the scrotum develops rugae as the fetus matures.
  - Female genitalia: Initially, the female fetus has a large clitoris and small labia majora. As the fetus matures, the labia majora enlarge, while the clitoris shrinks.

Infants born at 24 to 25 weeks

The modified Ballard score is used to accurately determine the gestational age of extremely premature infants. Infants born at 24 to 25 weeks gestational age will have:

- Skin - Very thin with visible veins. Absent or minimal vernix caseosa as it is just beginning to be secreted at 2 weeks.
- Lanugo - Sparse.
- Feet - Smooth plantar surfaces or faint marks on the anterior surfaces.
- Areolae - Newly developing, breast bud not yet present.
- Eyes - Open.
- Ears - No or very limited recoil.
- Posture - Immature, indicated by limited flexion of the limbs while infant is in supine position.
- Square window sign - Shows decreased flexion at the wrist of approximately 60° to 90°.
- Range of motion - Increased ROM (lone tone) when performing the popliteal angle, scarf sign, and heel to ear examinations.
- Arm recoil - Limited or no recoil.

Full-term (40-week) infant

Neuromuscular characteristics of a full-term (40-week) infant are as follows:

- Supine resting posture - Hips, knees, and arms all flexed past 90°, indicating mature muscular tone.
- Square window - The wrist flexes to 0°, reflecting very little resistance to the extensor muscles of the wrist.
- Arm recoil - Arms recoil past 90°. Contact between the infant's fist and face demonstrates mature tone in the bicep muscles.
- Popliteal angle - < 90° knee flexion.

- Scarf sign - The arms cannot be drawn past the ipsilateral axillary line because of the mature tone of the posterior shoulder girdle flexor muscles.
- Heel to ear - Resistance is felt in the knee and hip when the heel is at the femoral crease because of the tone of the posterior pelvic girdle flexor muscles.

SGA

Small for gestational age (SGA) infants are those whose weight places them below the 10th percentile for their gestational age. SGA is also called dysmaturity and intrauterine growth restriction. SGA babies commonly aspirate meconium and have a low Apgar score, asphyxia, hypoglycemia, and polycythemia. Common causes of SGA include:
- Multiple gestations (twins, triplets, quadruplets)
- Constitutional SGA because both parents are small
- Many genetic defects, such as trisomy 18 (Edwards syndrome), Down syndrome, and Turner syndrome
- Placental malfunction or misplacement (inadequate fetal nutrition from reduced blood flow, sepsis, placenta previa, or abruptio placentae)
- Maternal disease (preeclampsia; high blood pressure; malnutrition; advanced diabetes mellitus; chronic kidney, heart, or respiratory disease; and anemia)
- Infections such as cytomegalovirus, toxoplasmosis, and rubella
- Maternal tobacco, illegal drug, or alcohol use during pregnancy
- Birth defects

LGA

Large for gestational age (LGA) infants are those whose weight places them above the 90th percentile for their gestational age. The main pathologic cause for LGA is maternal diabetes (either gestational diabetes or diabetes mellitus). Infants exposed to elevated levels of glucose produce elevated amounts of insulin, which has an anabolic effect on the developing fetus, causing macrosomia (large body). Poor control of diabetes during pregnancy generally results in a larger infant with these common health problems:
- Delivery complications (shoulder dystocia, clavicle fracture, prolonged vaginal exit requiring use of forceps or cesarean delivery, and perinatal asphyxia)
- Abnormal blood test results (hypoglycemia developing within 1 to 2 hours of birth, hyperbilirubinemia, hypocalcemia, hypomagnesemia, hyperviscosity [thickened blood] secondary to polycythemia [elevated platelets])
- Jaundice
- Feeding intolerance
- Lethargy
- Respiratory distress
- Birth defects

Newborn skin

Newborns' skin appearance depends on the development and thickening of their dermis, epidermis, and vernix caseosa. When skin develops during week 15 of gestation, it is initially thin and translucent. By week 20, vernix caseosa production begins. Vernix is a thick, waxy substance secreted by the sebaceous glands and mixed with sloughed-off skin cells, often described as "cheesy." The stratum corneum (protective top layer of the epidermis) develops from weeks 20 to 24. The epidermis continues to develop and thicken, and is able to form a water barrier by week 32. Near term, the vernix washes away and the skin becomes more wrinkled without its protection. The skin's appearance at different gestational ages are explained as follows:

- 24 to 26 weeks - Translucent, red, many visible blood vessels, and scant vernix.
- 35 to 40 weeks - Deep cracks, no visible blood vessels, and thick vernix.
- 42 to 44 weeks - Dry, peeling skin, no vernix, and loss of subcutaneous fat.

Neonatal reflexes

Neonatal reflexes are explained as follows:

- Palmar grasping – To elicit the reflex stroke the infant's palm. The infant responds by grasping your finger. Grasp reflex is stronger in premature infants and fades away at 2 to 3 months of age. Absence indicates CNS deficit or muscle injury.
- Rooting – To elicit the reflex stroke the side of the infant's cheek. The infant turns his/her head in the same direction as your touch, and opens his/her mouth to feed. Rooting reflex helps the infant find and latch onto his/her mother's breast.
- Sucking – To elicit the reflex touch the infant's mouth. The infant sucks. Premature infants may have an absent or weak suck reflex, as it usually develops around week 32 of gestation. Weak or absent reflex indicates CNS deficit or depression.
- Moro (startle) – To elicit the reflex make a loud sound or give the infant a gentle jolt. The infant extends his/her arms, legs, and neck, and then pulls back his/her arms and legs. He/she may also cry. Moro reflex disappears at 5 to 6 months of age. Asymmetric response indicates peripheral nerve injury, fractures (long bones, clavicle, or skull).
- Blinking – To elicit the reflex flash light at eyes. Eyelids close. Absence or delay may indicate cerebral palsy, hydrocephalus, and developmental delay.
- Tonic neck (fencing) – To elicit the reflex, with infant supine, turn head to one side. Extremities flex on opposite side and extend on same side. May be incomplete immediately after birth and should diminish by 4 months. Persistence > 4 months may indicate neurological abnormalities.
- Babinski (plantar) – To elicit the reflex stroke the lateral aspect of the sole from heel to ball of foot. Hyperextension of all toes. Persists until ≤ 2 years after which the toes flex.
- Trunk incurvation (Galant) – To elicit the reflex, with infant prone, stroke down one side of the spine (1 inch from spine). Pelvis turns to stimulated side. Absence indicates CNS depression or lesion of spinal cord. Should disappear by 4 months.
- Tongue extrusion – To elicit the reflex touch tip of tongue. Neonate pushes tongue out of mouth. Continuous or repetitive extrusion indicates CNS abnormalities or seizure activity.

Jitteriness

Jitteriness (tremor of chin and extremities) occurs in about half of neonates within the first few days of life and may persist intermittently when the infant is excited or crying for 2 months or less. Jitteriness may also be present with drug withdrawal, hypoglycemia, hypocalcemia, and encephalopathy. Jitteriness must be differentiated from seizures, which may have a similar appearance.

Characteristics of jitteriness include:
- Lack of ocular deviations or other abnormalities
- Gentle restraint halts jitteriness
- Stimulation elicits jitteriness
- Clonic jerking has both fast and slow elements
- Autonomic changes involving the heart rate, respirations, and blood pressure are not present.
- EEG is normal

Jitteriness is distinct from shuddering, a 10- to 15-second period of fast tremors that may recur 100 times or less daily. Both jitteriness and shuddering are benign findings that require no treatment.

Weight, measurements, and vital signs

Neonatal appearance, measurements, and vital signs should be as follows:
- Head - Disproportionately large for body.
- Body – Long.
- Extremities - Short and in flexed position. (Feet usually dorsiflexed after breech birth.)
- Hands – Clenched.
- Neck - Short and chin resting on chest
- Abdomen – Prominent
- Hips – Narrow
- Chest – Rounded
- Weight - 2,500 to 4,000 g (average about 3,400). Physiologic weight loss is 5% to 10% for full term and 155 for preterm.
- Length - 45 to 55 cm (average 50 cm).
- Head circumference - 32 to 38 cm (usually 2 cm greater than chest circumference)
- Chest circumference - 30 to 36 cm
- Temperature - Temperature drops rapidly (skin temperature falls 0.3°C/minute) after birth with exposure to ambient room temperature but stabilizes within 8 to 12 hours. Temperature is usually measured by axillary method (for 3 minutes) and ranges from 36.3° to 37°C.
- Blood pressure - 56 to 77/33 to 50 mm Hg
- Pulse - 120 to 150 bpm awake; 100 bpm asleep; 180 bmp crying
- Respiration - 30-60 per minute

Brazelton Neonatal Behavioral Assessment Scale

The Brazelton Neonatal Behavioral Assessment Scale is a multidimensional scale that is used to assess a neonate's state, temperament, and behavioral patterns. It includes assessment of 18 reflexes, 28 behaviors, and 6 other characteristics. It is usually completed on day 3 with an attempt to elicit the most positive response, usually when the infant is comforted and in a quiet, dim room. Scoring correlates to the child's awake or sleep state. Infants are scored according to response in many areas, including:
- Habituation: Ability to diminish response to repeat stimuli
- Visual and auditory orientation: Ability to respond to stimuli, fixate, and follow a visual object

- Motor activity: Assessment of body tone in various activities
- Variations: Changes in color, state, activity, alertness, and excitement during the exam
- Self-quieting activities: Frequency and speed of self-calming activities, such as sucking on hand, putting hand to mouth, focusing on object or sound
- Social behaviors: Ability to cuddle, engage, and enjoy physical contact

Awake states

Infants have different levels of consciousness in the 4 awake states. Infants respond differently to outside stimuli and interaction from caregivers, depending on which state they are in:
- Drowsy: This is characterized by variable activity, mild startles, and smooth movement. There is some facial movement. Eyes open and close, breathing is irregular, and response to stimuli may be delayed.
- Quiet alert: The infant rarely moves, breathing is regular, and the infant focuses intently on individuals or objects that are within focal range, widening eyes. Face appears bright and alert, breathing is regular, and the infant focuses on stimuli.
- Active alert: The infant moves frequently and has much facial movement, although face not as bright and alert, eyes may have a dull glaze, breathing is irregular, and there are variable responses to outside stimuli.
- Crying: Characterized by grimacing, eyes shut, irregular breathing, increased movement with color changes, and marked response to both internal and external stimuli.

Sleep
Infants spend a high percentage of their time in sleep states. Sleep periods are divided into active sleep or quiet sleep by observing the infant's behavior:
- Quiet sleep is restorative and fosters anabolic growth. Quiet sleep is associated with increased cell mitosis and replication, lowered oxygen consumption, and the release of growth hormone. During quiet sleep, the infant appears relaxed, moves minimally, and breathes smoothly and regularly. The eyelids are still. The infant only responds to intense stimuli during quiet sleep
- Active sleep is associated with processing and storing of information. Rapid eye movement (REM) occurs during active sleep, but it is unknown if newborn infants are able to dream. During active sleep, the infant moves occasionally and breathes irregularly. Eye movements can be seen beneath the eyelids. Infants spend most of their sleep time in active sleep, and it usually precedes wakening

Muscle tone

Determining the quality of muscle tone in a neonate is an important part of neuromuscular assessment. The child is placed supine with the head in neutral position and the NNP moves body parts (arms, legs, head) to determine if the muscle tone is flaccid, jittery, or hypertonic. Neonates are slightly hypertonic so that some resistance should be felt to movement, such as when moving a leg or straightening an arm. Tone should be symmetric. The extremities are usually flexed and legs abducted to abdomen. This assessment allows the NNP to differentiate common fine tremors or jitteriness found in neonates from seizure activity or nervous system disorders that cause muscular twitching. Normal fine tremors are usually halted by holding or flexing the extremity while seizure activity or twitching does not resolve by holding.

Routine nursing care

Screening of the newborn to detect genetic diseases varies somewhat from one state to another. Because about 1 in 200 newborns has chromosomal abnormalities, screening is an important tool. However, many birth defects are not genetic in origin, such as defects caused by maternal alcohol abuse or vitamin deficiency. Screening tests include the following:

- Biotinidase deficiency (autosomal recessive)
- Congenital adrenal hyperplasia (autosomal recessive)
- Congenital hearing loss (autosomal recessive, autosomal dominant, or mitochondrial)
- Congenital hypothyroidism (autosomal recessive or autosomal dominant)
- Cystic fibrosis (autosomal recessive)
- Galactosemia (autosomal recessive)
- Homocystinuria (autosomal recessive)
- Maple syrup urine disease (autosomal recessive)
- Medium-chain acyl-coenzyme A dehydrogenase (autosomal recessive)
- Phenylketonuria (autosomal recessive)
- Sickle cell disease (autosomal recessive)
- Tyrosinemia (2 types are autosomal recessive; third type is unclear)

Eye prophylaxis

Most states mandate eye prophylaxis for the newborn, although a number of studies suggest that parents can safely choose to refuse this prophylaxis if the mother has had prenatal care and screening for STDs. However, most pediatricians still support prophylaxis. Medications used for prophylaxis include erythromycin eye ointment, tetracycline eye ointment, or 1% silver nitrate drops. Erythromycin is usually the drug of choice because it is active against both gonococcal and chlamydial infections. Silver nitrate is rarely used now even though it is effective because it can cause eye irritation. Ointment should be applied to the inside of the lower lids (inner canthus to outer) and the eyes then closed to help to spread the ointment. Excess ointment can be gently wiped from the eyes after 1 minute.

Thermoregulation

At delivery, minimize heat loss while evaluating the newborn by following these steps:
- Dry the infant thoroughly (including hair) to minimize evaporative heat loss, and remove wet towels
- Place a cap on the infant's head, as the head is the most significant area of heat loss
- When the infant is to be weighed, cover the scales with a warm cloth to minimize conductive heat loss
- Place infant in a warm environment, such as:
  o Skin-to-skin contact with mother, and cover them with a warm blanket
  o Bundled in warm blankets and given to mother to hold
  o Underneath a preheated warmer for further evaluation or resuscitation

Minimizing heat loss is especially important if the newborn is premature or has intrauterine growth restriction, but full-term newborns also suffer if they become chilled.

Skin temperature probes

Skin temperature probes are often used to monitor the temperature of the infant in an Isolette or radiant warmer. Incorrect placement of the probe can alter the reading, causing the warming device to deliver too much or too little heat. The temperature probe should not be placed over a bony area of the body or over an area where brown adipose tissue is abundant. Brown adipose tissue is abundant around the neck, the midscapular region of the back, the mediastinum, and organs in the thoracic cavity, kidneys, and adrenal glands. A common probe placement area for an infant who is supine is over the liver. If the probe is not making good skin contact, it will indicate that the infant is cold, and the warmer will deliver increased amounts of heat, possibly causing hyperthermia. If the probe is underneath the infant, it may indicate an artificially warm temperature and decrease heat to the infant, causing hypothermia.

NTE

A neutral thermal environment (NTE) is a place in which the infant's body temperature is maintained within a normal range without alterations in metabolic rate or increased oxygen consumption (i.e., environmental temperature in which oxygen consumption and glucose consumption are lowest). Infants who are in an NTE are not utilizing energy to maintain their body temperature in the normal range. Just because an infant has a normal body temperature does not mean he/she is in an NTE. The infant may still be utilizing mechanisms, such as non-shivering thermogenesis, to maintain body temperatures, as evidenced by increased oxygen consumption and poor weight gain over time. Charts are commercially available that outline the appropriate NTE for infants based on current weight and birth weight.

Radiant warmers

Radiant warmers are devices that provide overhead heat directly to the infant. Radiant heaters provide an area for direct observation and free access to the infant, which is very useful in the initial evaluation and resuscitation (if necessary) of the newborn, or for procedures such as intubation or line placement. Radiant heat devices work best if the room temperature is kept above 25°C. Two problems related to radiant warmers include:
- Promote dehydration if an infant is placed under them for a prolonged amount of time, especially if the infant is premature
- Risk overheating the infant or cause first-degree burns

Temperature sensors must be appropriately placed and the infant's temperature monitored frequently to ensure the infant is not being over- or under-heated.

Circumcision

Circumcision is surgical removal of the foreskin of the penis. Circumcision has decreased in popularity in the United States over the past 20 years, with current rates at approximately 50%. Controversies exist concerning the need for circumcision:
- Minimal advantages:
  - Decreased incidence of phimosis and urinary tract infections.
  - Decreased risk for penile cancer and the contraction of sexually transmitted diseases in the adult.
- Risks:
  - Bleeding
  - Infection
  - Pain unrelieved by anesthetic
  - Decreased sexual sensitivity in the adult
  - Permanent damage to the urinary tract and sex organs necessitating reconstructive surgery

Local anesthesia or nerve block should be used to prevent pain during the procedure. If the Plastibell is used, the plastic rim stays in place 3 to 4 days until healing. The rim usually falls off but may be removed if still in place in 8 days. For other procedures, the glans is usually covered with petrolatum gauze for the first few days to promote healing and prevent irritation.

Complications of the Neonatal Period

AOP

Premature infants (especially those younger than 34 weeks) often exhibit apnea of prematurity (AOP). AOP begins at birth and is believed to be caused by immaturity of the nervous system, improving as the brain matures. It may persist for a 4 to 8 weeks. There are 3 types of apnea:
- Central: no airflow or effort to breathe
- Obstructive: no airflow, but effort to breathe
- Mixed: both central and obstructive elements (75% of AOP)

Symptoms include:
- Swallowing during apneic periods.
- Apnea >20 seconds.
- Apnea < 20 seconds with bradycardia 30 beats < normal.
- Oxygen saturation < 85% persisting ≥ 5 seconds.
- Cyanosis.

Treatment includes:
- Tactile stimulation (rubbing limbs or thorax or gently slapping bottoms of feet) or gently lifting the jaw to relieve obstruction.
- Oxygen or bag/mask ventilation for bradycardia and decreased oxygen saturation.
- Continuous positive airway pressure (CPAP) for mixed or obstructive apnea.
- Aminophylline/theophylline or caffeine (for central apnea) may increase contractions of diaphragm.

Birth asphyxia

Birth asphyxia is the cause of many problems after birth. Birth asphyxia is defined as an event that alters the exchange of gas (oxygen and carbon dioxide). This interference with gas exchange leads to a decrease in the amount of oxygen delivered to the fetus along with an increase in the level of carbon dioxide the fetus is exposed to. This gas imbalance causes the fetus to switch from normal aerobic metabolism to anaerobic metabolism. Fetal distress results and this distress then leads to increased fetal heart rate, release of meconium into the amniotic fluid, and lowered pH. Infants experiencing birth asphyxia will often present at birth with Apgar scores that are less than 5. Symptoms of birth asphyxia are as follows:

- Mild:
  - Overly alert for the first 45 minutes to 1 hour following birth (infants are normally sleepy after about 15 minutes following birth).
  - The pupils are dilated.
  - The respiratory rate and the heart rate will both be slightly increased.
  - Newborn reflexes and muscle tone are normal.
  - Oxygen may be administered.
- Moderate:
  - Hypothermia as evidenced by low body temperature.
  - Hypoglycemia as glucose stores are used up trying to supply organs needed energy
  - Pupils are constricted
  - Signs of respiratory distress are evident
  - May experience seizure activity at 12 to 24 hours of age
  - Lethargy (floppy infant)
  - Bradycardia
- Severe: This requires close monitoring in a NICU.
  - Pale color related to the inability of the heart to perfuse the body
  - Cerebral edema related to apnea episodes and/or intracranial hemorrhage

Resuscitation will vary according to the infant's condition, but warming the infant, stabilizing the glucose level, and providing oxygen or extracorporeal membrane oxygenation (EMCO) (in severe cases) may be indicated.

TTN

Transient tachypnea of newborn (TTN) occurs when fluid in the lungs is not adequately absorbed after birth. The neonate usually exhibits symptoms within 36 hours of birth and the condition typically resolves within 3 days. TTN is most common in infants delivered by cesarean, but premature birth and mothers who smoke or have diabetes increase risk to infant.

Symptoms include:
- Dyspnea (> 60/min)
- Sternal retraction (mild)
- Expiratory grunt
- Nasal flaring
- Poor feeding (because of increased respiratory rate)

Laboratory findings:
- ABGs: Hypoxemia
- Chest radiograph: Fluid in lungs

Treatment includes:
- Monitor oxygen saturation levels
- Provide supplemental oxygen as indicated
- Provide IV fluids or nasogastric feedings if unable to take oral feedings

MAS

Meconium aspiration syndrome (MAS) occurs when meconium expelled in the amniotic fluid (occurring in about 20% of pregnancies) is aspirated before, during, or after birth. Blood and amniotic fluids may be aspirated as well. Some infants may present with symptoms at birth, but sometimes symptoms are delayed for a number of hours. Symptoms are similar to TTN but more severe, and the infant appears more compromised.

Symptoms include:
- Tachypnea with prolonged expirations.
- Nasal flaring and sternal retraction, course crackles, lethargy, hypoxemia, hypercapnia, cyanosis, metabolic and respiratory acidosis (PaO_2 decreased even with 100% oxygen).
- Hyperventilation may occur initially with hypoventilation later.
- Chest x-rays may show infiltrates atelectasis, and hypoinflated areas as well as hyperinflated areas, pulmonary hypertension, hypothermia, hypoglycemia.
- Long-term sequelae may include airway obstruction, hyperinflation, and exercise-induced bronchospasm.

Treatment includes:
- Preventive suctioning of the oropharynx as the head is delivered.
- Tracheal/bronchial suctioning to remove meconium plugs as indicated.
- Umbilical (arterial and venous) monitoring of ABGs, IV fluids, intubation, oxygen, assisted ventilation (CPAP at 5 to 7 cm H2O), and suctioning of the trachea for infants with respiratory distress (weak respirations', bradycardia, hypotonia).
- EMCO as indicated.
- Nitric oxide if persistent pulmonary hypertension of newborn (PPHN) occurs.
- Antibiotic prophylaxis to prevent pneumonia.
- Thermoregulation.
- Surfactant.

Neonatal jaundice

Jaundice is yellowing of the skin and sclera (whites of the eyes), indicating elevated bilirubin levels (hyperbilirubinemia). Elevated bilirubin levels occur normally during the newborn period because of the rapid breakdown of fetal hemoglobin after birth and the immaturity of enzymatic pathways in the newborn's liver (the organ responsible for metabolizing bilirubin). Physiological jaundice describes this normal process, which usually becomes evident on the second or third day of life by yellowing of the face. As bilirubin levels increase, the trunk and extremities become involved, and the skin yellows. The baby's eyes are covered and the baby placed in under blue lights (phototherapy). For most infants, jaundice is transient and resolves within a few days. Persistent or pronounced jaundice may indicate that further diagnostic testing or intervention is needed.

Hyperbilirubinemia

Hyperbilirubinemia, excess of bilirubin in the blood, is characterized by jaundice. Hyperbilirubinemia is evaluated according to the levels of direct (conjugated) bilirubin and/or indirect (unconjugated) bilirubin:

- Direct/conjugated bilirubin levels increase with blockage of bile ducts, hepatitis, or other liver damage, including drug reaction.
- Indirect/unconjugated bilirubin levels increase with anemias (such as hemolytic disorders) and transfusion reactions.

Basic types of hyperbilirubinemia are:

- Physiologic - Common in newborns and usually benign, resulting from immature hepatic function and increased RBC hemolysis. Infants have larger red blood cells with a shorter life than adults, leading to more RBC destruction and resulting in an increased load of serum bilirubin, which the liver of the newborn cannot handle. Premature infants have an even greater physiologic jaundice as their RBCs live even shorter lives than the term infant's. Onset is usually within 24 to 48 hours, peaking in 72 hours for full-term or 5 days for preterm infants and declining within a week. Phototherapy is the indicated treatment for total serum bilirubin ≥ 18 mg/dL.
- Hemolytic - Caused by blood/antigen (Rh) incompatibility with onset in first 24 hours. Preventive treatment is RhoGAM prenatally or postnatal exchange transfusion. This type of hyperbilirubinemia may also result from ABO incompatibility, but rarely requires treatment other than phototherapy.
- Breast-feeding associated - Relates to inadequate calories during early breastfeeding with onset of 2 to 3 days. This slows the excretion of stool and allows bilirubin levels to rise. More frequent feeding with caloric supplements is usually sufficient, but phototherapy may be used for bilirubin 18 to 20 mg/dL.
- Breast milk jaundice - May result from breast milk breaking down bilirubin and its being reabsorbed in the gut. Characterized by less frequent stools and onset in 4th to 5th day, peaking in 10 to 15 days; jaundice may persist for a number of weeks. Treatment involves discontinuing breastfeeding for 24 hours.

Indications for phototherapy and exchange transfusion

Phototherapy is often used to treat hyperbilirubinemia to prevent the need for exchange transfusion. For phototherapy, the infant is placed under special lights (15 to 20 cm above the infant) that will decrease the bilirubin levels in the blood. Indications include:

- Weight: 500 to 750 g/Serum bilirubin level: 5 to 8 mg/dL
- Weight: 751 to 1,000 g/ Serum bilirubin level: 6 to 10 mg/dL
- Weight: 1,001 to 1,250 g/ Serum bilirubin level: 8 to 10 mg/dL
- Weight: 1,251 to 1,500 g /Serum bilirubin level: 10 to 12 mg dL

Exchange transfusions may be used for hyperbilirubinemia. Blood less than 72 hours old is used to maintain potassium levels. Indications include:
- Weight: 500 to 750 g/ Serum bilirubin level: 12 to 15 mg/dL
- Weight: 751 to 1,000 g/ Serum bilirubin level: > 15 mg/dL
- Weight: 1,001 to 1,250 g/ Serum bilirubin level: 15 to 18 mg/dL
- Weight: 1,251 to 1,500 g/ Serum bilirubin level: 17 to 20 mg/dL

There are many risks associated with exchange transfusions, including vascular complications, such as emboli or thrombosis, often related to umbilical catheters. Cardiac complications include dysrhythmias and overload, leading to arrest. Clotting disorders may result from over-heparinization (reversed with protamine sulfate). Electrolyte and glucose abnormalities as well as infection may occur.

HDN

Rh sensitivity may occur when an Rh-negative mother's blood contacts blood of an Rh-positive fetus, causing the mother's immune system to make antibodies that can cross the placenta and attack the fetal Rh-positive red blood cells, resulting in hemolytic disease of the newborn (HDN). This is primarily a problem during second or subsequent pregnancies. In the fetus, hemolysis triggers increased RBC production (erythroblastosis fetalis), a form of anemia that left untreated results in severe/fatal edema (hydrops fetalis) that can cause congestive heart failure. Erythroblastosis fetalis is characterized by jaundice, fever, generalized edema, cyanosis, and hepatosplenomegaly. Hyperbilirubinemia and jaundice associated with HDN occur from RBC destruction, leading to neurological impairment (kernicterus). Treatment includes exchange transfusion in utero or after birth. Management of fetal hemolysis may include early delivery (at least 32 weeks after confirmation of pulmonary maturity if possible), with risks associated with prematurity, and intrauterine transfusion, which can cause fetal distress, hematoma, maternal-fetal hemorrhage, and fetal death (10% to 20%).

CHEAP TORCHES and TORCH panel

CHEAP TORCHES is the acronym used to recall common causes of congenital and neonatal infections. Many congenital infections are present for at least a month prior to birth and remain present at birth:
C Chickenpox (varicella) **H** Hepatitis (B, C, and E) **E** Enterovirus (RNA viruses, including coxsackievirus, echovirus, and poliovirus) **A** AIDS (HIV) **P** Parvovirus (B 19)

T Toxoplasmosis **O** Other (group B streptococcus, Candida, Listeria, TB, lymphocytic choriomeningitis) **R** Rubella (measles) **C** Cytomegalovirus **H** Herpes simplex virus
E Every other STD (Chlamydia, gonorrhea, Ureaplasma, papillomavirus **S** Syphilis Exposure to these pathogens in utero may cause a miscarriage or congenital defect, especially if the exposure was during the first trimester. Symptoms may include small for gestational age, enlarged liver and spleen, thrombocytopenia, skin rash, jaundice, seizures, or encephalitis. The TORCH panel, which tests for toxoplasmosis, rubella, cytomegalovirus, and herpes simplex virus, is commonly used to screen pregnant women for infectious diseases.

Sepsis

Neonatal sepsis is a particular risk for preterm infants < 1,000 g and may be associated with a wide range of pathogens, both bacterial and viral. Early onset (≤ 72 hours) is usually related to maternal transmission and late onset (4 to 90 days) to invasive devices. Early-onset sepsis most often is characterized by pneumonia and late-onset by bacteremia and/or meningitis. Symptoms vary according to pathogen, onset, and primary site of infection:

- Nonspecific signs of respiratory distress, CNS irritation, and metabolic disorders
- Pneumonia: Tachypnea, sternal retraction, grunting respirations, cyanosis, and apneic periods.
- Meningitis: Stupor, irritability, indications of increasing ICP, bulging anterior fontanel (but signs may be subtle in the neonate)
- Decreased cardiac output with pulmonary hypertension, signs of shock
- Hypo- or hyperglycemia, metabolic acidosis
- Jaundice
- DIC
- Necrotizing enterocolitis

Laboratory findings vary:

- Chest radiograph may show pneumonia
- CT/MRI may show abscesses, obstructive hydrocephalus
- Ultrasound may show abnormalities of ventricles and brain structures (meningitis)
- Thrombocytopenia < 100,000/mcL
- WBC counts may not be elevated and may not show shift to left, especially initially
- Immature to total neutrophil ratio increased
- Clotting abnormalities (with DIC)
- Culture and sensitivities may not show infection because of small sample size
- CSF: Elevated WBC count and protein level and positive culture (with meningitis)
- Increased C-reactive protein

Treatment includes:

- IV antibiotics: Aminoglycoside and expanded-spectrum penicillin most common but vancomycin or oxacillin may be used for hospital-acquired infection
- Surgical incision and drainage of abscess
- Ventriculoperitoneal shunt for hydronephrosis related to meningitis
- NPO initially and then enteral feedings or TPN
- Thermoregulation as indicated (radiant warmer, incubator)
- Maintenance of fluid balance and IV fluids as needed
- Intubation/ventilation as needed

Bacterial meningitis

Bacterial meningitis may manifest differently, depending on the age of the infant:

- Early onset: The infant may exhibit signs of shock within 24 hours of birth with rapid progression of symptoms that include respiratory distress with episodes of apnea, hypotension, thermodysregulation, inconsolable crying, seizures, diarrhea, jaundice, and hepatomegaly

- Late onset: Symptoms may be very nonspecific and can include weight loss, hypo- or hyperthermia, jaundice, irritability, lethargy, and irregular respirations with periods of apnea. More specific signs may include increasing signs of illness, difficulty feeding with loss of suck reflex, hypotonia, posturing, weak cry, seizures, and bulging fontanels (may be a late sign). Nuchal rigidity does not usually occur with neonates but may be a late sign

Treatment includes antibiotic therapy as indicated according to cultures and sensitivities. Initial therapy usually includes ampicillin or penicillin G and an aminoglycoside. Treatment is monitored by examination of CSF with treatment usually for 2 weeks after CSF becomes sterile. Kernig sign and Brudzinski sign are generally absent in neonates.

Ophthalmia neonatorum

Conjunctivitis is inflammation of the conjunctiva of the eye from bacteria, viruses, or chemical irritants. If infectious conjunctivitis occurs less than 30 days from birth, it is referred to as ophthalmia neonatorum and is commonly acquired during delivery:
- Pathogenic agents include Chlamydia trachomatis, Neisseria gonorrhoeae, and herpesvirus. It can also be caused by chemical irritants, such as silver nitrate (the reason it is no longer routinely used for eye prophylaxis)
- Antibiotic drops or ointment (typically erythromycin ointment) is applied to the newborns eyes to prevent conjunctivitis. Intravenous acyclovir is given to infants exposed to herpesvirus

Untreated, gonococcal conjunctivitis usually develops in 5 days or less of birth and is characterized by purulent discharge and inflammation. It is treated with IV antibiotics (benzylpenicillin or cefotaxime). Chlamydial conjunctivitis develops at 3 to 14 days and is characterized by watery discharge and less inflammation than gonococcal conjunctivitis. It is treated with IV erythromycin and topical tetracycline.

STDs that cause infection in the neonate

Maternal sexually transmitted diseases can cause infection in the neonate. Common STDs include:
- Chlamydia: Infants most commonly exhibit conjunctivitis
- Gonorrhea: Infants exposed to Neisseria gonorrhoeae during vaginal delivery most commonly develop bilateral conjunctivitis (ophthalmia neonatorum) if left untreated. In some cases, disseminated gonococcal infection (DGI) can occur in infants
- Syphilis: Infants may be asymptomatic, even with full-system infection. Multiple system disorders and abnormalities can occur, including nonviral hepatitis with jaundice, hepatosplenomegaly, pseudoparalysis, pneumonitis, bone marrow failure, myocarditis, meningitis, anemia, edema associated with nephritic syndrome, and a rash on the palms of the hands and soles of the feet
- Herpes: Localized lesions may occur at 10 to 12 days. Disseminated infection may cause pneumonitis, hepatitis, and encephalitis
- HIV/AIDS: Infants are asymptomatic at birth and may test falsely positive
- Trichomoniasis: Infants may be born preterm and with low birth weight
- (less than 2,500 g)

Neonatal pneumonia

Neonatal pneumonia may result from an intrauterine infection (transplacental, aspiration of meconium, or infected amniotic fluid) or neonatal infection acquired during hospitalization after delivery. Premature infants are at increased risk. Common bacterial agents include *E. coli*, *Klebsiella*, *S. aureus*, group B streptococcus, *Pseudomonas,* and group A streptococci. Common viral agents include herpes simplex, cytomegalovirus, varicella, RSV, parainfluenza, enterovirus, and adenovirus. Symptoms are similar to respiratory distress and sepsis:

- Tachypnea with diminished breath sounds and rales
- Expiratory grunting
- Sternal retraction
- Cyanosis
- Hypoxemia and hypercapnia
- Hypoglycemia
- Shock
- Chest x-ray: Similar to RDS

Treatment includes:

- Administer antibiotics (ampicillin with an aminoglycoside initially for bacterial infection), usually for 10 to 14 days
- Provide thermoregulation
- Maintain blood glucose levels
- Provide supplementary oxygen and assisted ventilation as necessary
- Treat acidosis (respiratory and/or metabolic)
- IV fluids
- Monitor for evidence of DIC

Neonatal bowel obstructions

Bowel obstruction occurs when there is a mechanical obstruction of the passage of intestinal contents because of constriction of the lumen, occlusion of the lumen, or lack of muscular contractions (paralytic ileus). Obstruction may be caused by congenital or acquired abnormalities/disorders:

- Small Bowel Obstructions:
  - Duodenal atresia
  - Malrotation and volvulus
  - Jejunoileal atresia
  - Meconium ileus
  - Meconium peritonitis
- Large Bowel Obstructions:
  - Hirschsprung disease
  - Anorectal malformations
  - Meconium plug syndrome

Symptoms include:
- Abdominal pain, distention, and rigidity
- Vomiting and dehydration
- Diminished or no bowel sounds
- Severe constipation (obstipation)
- Respiratory distress from diaphragm pushing against pleural cavity
- Shock as plasma volume diminishes and electrolytes enter intestines from bloodstream
- Sepsis as bacteria proliferates in bowel and invade bloodstream

Hypertrophic pyloric stenosis

Hypertrophic pyloric stenosis (PS) is obstruction of the pyloric sphincter between the gastric pylorus and small intestine, caused by hypertrophy and hyperplasia of the circular muscle of the pylorus so the enlarged tissue obstructs the sphincter. PS is more common in boys than girls and has a genetic predisposition. Onset of symptoms is usually more than 3 weeks:
- Projectile vomiting (1 to 4 feet) usually shortly after eating but may be delayed for a few hours. Emesis may be blood-tinged but nonbilious
- Infant is hungry and eats readily, but shows weight loss and signs of dehydration
- Upper abdominal distention with palpable mass in epigastrium (to right of umbilicus).
- Visible left to right peristaltic waves

Diagnosis is based on ultrasound. Decreased sodium and potassium levels may not be evident with dehydration.   Treatment consists of:
 IV fluids to restore hydration and electrolyte balance.
Surgical pyloromyotomy: longitudinal incisions through the circular muscle fibers down to the submucosa to release the restriction and allow the muscle to expand.

Intestinal atresia

When a portion of the bowel comes to a stop and then starts back up again forming a discontinuous or segmented bowel, this is called intestinal atresia. This condition usually relates to failures during the 5th to 10th week of fetal development, so it is often associated with other anomalies. The most common site for atresia to occur in the neonate is the duodenum. Atresia can also occur in the ileum, jejunum, colon, and rarely the stomach. An atresia that occurs anywhere in the intestine except the duodenum is not associated with any other disorders. However, an atresia that occurs in the duodenum (the most common type) may be (30% of the time) associated with other disorders such as trisomy 21, congenital heart disease, and VACTERL association. The only treatment for intestinal atresia is surgical reconnection of the bowel.

Imperforate anus

Imperforate anus (anorectal malfunction) is diagnosed by physical examination, digital or endoscopic examination, and contrast radiography with the infant inverted and an opaque marker at the anal dimple to outline the location of a pouch in relation to the normal position of the anus. Symptoms include:
- Absence of anal opening: No meconium in 24 to 48 hours, abdominal distention, and vomiting
- Rectovaginal fistula or rectourethral fistula: Symptoms may not be evident at first because stool passes through fistula
- Fistula between the rectum and the bladder: Gas or fecal material may be expelled through the urethra
- Displacement of the anus: Chronic constipation develops over time

Most forms require surgery, type depending upon extent of abnormality:
- Simple excision of anal opening may suffice
- 2- to 3-step procedures for higher anomalies in which a colostomy is first performed with later reconstruction of the anus in the proper position, involving anoplasty and pull-through procedures
- Manual dilation may treat stenosis

Meconium plug syndrome

Meconium plug syndrome (also called functional colonic obstruction) occurs when the first stool obstructs the intestinal tract and no other pathology is present. This will be evident in the first 24 to 48 hours of life, when the infant fails to pass the first meconium stool. Meconium plug syndrome usually occurs in full-term infants, infants of diabetic mothers, or infants with hypermagnesemia. The infant may have abdominal distension, poor feeding, and vomiting (often bilious in nature). An x-ray of the abdomen will show dilated loops of bowel. A contrast enema is diagnostic and helps differentiate from other causes of intestinal obstruction. It may also be therapeutic, causing the plug to pass. Infants usually do well after the plug has passed. A small percentage of infants initially identified as having meconium plug syndrome (5% to 10%) have Hirschsprung disease. The cause of meconium plug syndrome is thought to be immaturity of the ganglion cells of the colon.

CDH

Congenital diaphragmatic hernia (CDH) may cause severe respiratory distress. The primary CDHs that affect infants are posterolateral (Bochdalek):
- Left-sided (85%) includes herniation of the large and small intestine and intraabdominal organs into the thoracic cavity
- Right-sided (13%) may be asymptomatic or involve usually just the liver and part of the large intestine

Neonates with left CDH may exhibit severe respiratory distress and cyanosis. The lungs may be underdeveloped because of pressure exerted from displaced organs during fetal development. There may be a left hemithorax with a mediastinal shift and the heart pressing on the right lung, which may be hypoplastic. Bowel sounds are heard over the chest area. Pulmonary hypertension and cardiopulmonary failure may occur. Treatment includes:

- Immediate surgery repair
- High-frequency oscillation ventilation (HFOV) and nitric oxide for pulmonary hypoplasia.
- Extracorporeal membrane oxygenation (ECMO) for cardiopulmonary dysfunction

Despite treatment, mortality rates are 50%, and children who survive may have emphysema, with larger alveolar volume but inadequate numbers of alveoli.

Hirschsprung disease

Hirschsprung disease (congenital aganglionic megacolon) is failure of ganglion nerve cells to migrate to part of the bowel (usually the distal colon), so that part of the bowel lacks enervation and peristalsis, causing stool to accumulate and leading to distention and megacolon. There is a genetic predisposition to the disease that affects more males than females and is associated with trisomy 21 (Down syndrome). Symptoms include:

- Failure to pass meconium in 24 to 48 hours
- Poor feeding
- Bilious vomitus
- Abdominal distention

Delayed diagnosis:

- Chronic constipation
- Failure to thrive
- Periods of diarrhea and vomiting
- With infection: severe prostration with watery diarrhea, fever, hypotension

Treatment includes resection of aganglionic section and colorectal anastomosis. There are a number of procedures (Swenson, Duhamel, and Soave) but recently laparoscopic or transanal minimally invasive approaches have proven successful.

Malrotation/volvulus

When the intestines return to the abdominal cavity during the 10th to 12th week of fetal development, they undergo a rotation into their anatomically correct position. Sometimes this rotation fails, and the result is a malrotation. Malrotation is a congenital defect in which the intestines are attached to the back of the abdominal wall by one single attachment rather than a broad band of attachments across the abdomen, essentially suspending the bowels so that they can easily twist. This results in a volvulus (twisted bowel), cutting off blood supply. It may untwist but can lead to bowel infarction. Some children with malrotation have no symptoms, but most develop symptoms by 1 year:

- Cycles of cramping pain about every 15 to 30 minutes
- Abdominal distention
- Diarrhea, bloody stools, or no stools

- Vomiting (occurring soon after crying begins usually indicates small intestine obstruction; later vomiting usually indicates large intestine blockage)
- Tachycardia and tachypnea
- Decreased urinary output
- Fever

Treatment is by surgical repair.

Gastroschisis

Gastroschisis is extrusion of the nonrotated midgut through the abdominal wall to the right of umbilicus with no protective membrane covering matted, thickened loops of intestine. The abnormality is usually small, but the stomach and almost all of the small and large intestines can protrude. Because the intestines float without protection in amniotic fluid, there may be severe damage to the intestines with bowel atresia and ischemia. Gastroschisis is usually diagnosed with fetal ultrasound and is obvious at birth. These infants lose body temperature, fluids, and electrolytes, and receive IV fluids. The exposed organs are covered with sterile plastic film for protection and to prevent fluid loss, and a nasogastric feeding tube is inserted. Primary closure is done when the infant stabilizes for small abnormalities. Larger abnormalities may require stages with only part of organs returned to cavity and the remaining covered with a Silastic pouch until the abdominal cavity grows and surgical repair can be completed.

Omphalocele

Omphalocele is a congenital herniation of intestines or other organs through the base of the umbilicus with a protecting amniotic membrane but no skin. The sac may contain only a loop or most of bowel and the internal abdominal organs. This sac differentiates gastroschisis from omphalocele. *Diagnosis* is usually with fetal ultrasound. Symptoms vary widely. Maintaining integrity of tissues by keeping exposed sac or viscera moist and providing IV fluids are important. Small omphalocele are repaired immediately, but more extensive repair is usually delayed until the infant is stable if sac is intact. *Silvadene* cream toughens the sac, which is usually covered with a Silastic (plastic) pouch to protect the tissue. The abdomen may be unusually small, making correction difficult, so surgeons may wait 6 to 12 months while the abdominal cavity grows. Surgical repair may be done in stages over 8 to 10 days.

GER

Gastroesophageal reflux (GER) is involuntary regurgitation of stomach contents into the esophagus, usually caused by decreased tone in the lower esophageal sphincter in infants. GER *symptoms* include frequent nonbilious regurgitation, especially after feeding, usually not associated with respiratory distress, although some children may have colicky symptoms, and some may cough, choke, or wheeze, or have periods of apnea. Diagnosis is by upper GI contrast studies and pH probe study (the most diagnostic) performed over 12 to 24 hours. Treatment includes:
- Regulating feeding: Small, more frequent amounts, thickened with rice cereal
- Positioning: prone positioning after feeding/eating reduces regurgitation (although some concern remains about SIDS with infants). Placing infant in an upright position

(avoiding slumping) after meals or carrying the infant upright can help, but placing in infant seat may increase intraabdominal pressure
- Medications: Histamine-2 receptor blockers (ranitidine) or proton pump inhibitor (omeprazole), prokinetic agent (metoclopramide), and/or antacids (without aluminum).
- Surgery: Considered for severe or life-threatening symptoms

Acyanotic and cyanotic congenital heart disease

Congenital heart disease is one of the leading causes of death in children within the first year of life. There are two main types of congenital heart disease: acyanotic and cyanotic. They may also be classified according to hemodynamics related to the blood flow pattern:
- Cyanotic congenital defects:
  - Decreased pulmonary blood flow
    - Tetralogy of Fallot
    - Tricuspid atresia
  - Mixed blood flow
    - Hypoplastic left heart syndrome
    - Total anomalous pulmonary venous return
    - Transposition of great arteries
    - Truncus arteriosus.
    - Ebstein anomaly
- Acyanotic congenital defects:
  - Increased pulmonary blood flow
    - Atrial septal defect
    - Atrioventricular canal defect
    - Patent ductus arteriosus
    - Ventricular septal defect
  - Obstructed ventricular blood flow
    - Aortic stenosis
    - Coarctation of aorta
    - Pulmonic stenosis

TOF

Tetralogy of Fallot (TOF) is a combination of 4 different defects:
- Ventricular septal defect (usually with a large opening)
- Pulmonic stenosis with decreased blood flow to lungs
- Overriding aorta (displacement to the right so that it appears to come from both ventricles, usually overriding the ventricular septal defect), resulting in mixing of oxygenated and deoxygenated blood
- Right ventricular hypertrophy

Infants are often acutely cyanotic immediately after birth while others with less severe defects may have increasing cyanosis over the first year. Symptoms include:
- Intolerance to feeding or crying, resulting in increased cyanotic "blue spells" or "tet spells"
- Failure to thrive with poor growth
- Clubbing of fingers may occur over time

- Intolerance to activity as child grows
- Increased risk for emboli, brain attacks, brain abscess, seizures, fainting, or sudden death

Total surgical repair at 1 year or younger is now the preferred treatment rather than palliative procedures formerly used

Tricuspid atresia

Tricuspid atresia is lack of tricuspid valve between the right atrium and right ventricle so blood flows through the foramen ovale or an atrial defect to the left atrium and then through a ventricular wall defect from the left ventricle to the right ventricle and out to the lungs, causing oxygenated and deoxygenated bloods to mix. Pulmonic obstruction is common. Symptoms include:
- Cyanosis obvious postnatally
- Tachycardia and dyspnea
- Increasing hypoxemia and clubbing in older children
- Increased risk for bacterial endocarditis, brain abscess, and stroke

Treatment includes:
- Prostaglandin (alprostadil) to keep the ductus arteriosus and foramen ovale open if there are no septal defects
- Numerous surgical procedures, including pulmonary artery banding, shunting from the aorta to the pulmonary arteries, Glenn procedure (connecting superior vena cava to pulmonary artery to allow deoxygenated blood to flow to the lungs), atrial septostomy to enlarge the opening between the atria, and the Fontan corrective procedure (usually done at 2 to 4 years after previous stabilizing procedures)

HLHS

Hypoplastic left heart syndrome (HLHS) is underdevelopment of the left ventricle and ascending aortic atresia, causing inability of the heart to pump blood, so most blood flows from the left atrium through the foramen ovale to the right atrium and to the lungs with the descending aorta receiving blood through the ductus arteriosus. There may be valvular abnormalities as well. Mortality rates are 100% without surgical correction and 25% with correction. Symptoms may be mild until the ductus arteriosus closes at about 2 weeks, causing a marked increase in cyanosis and decreased cardiac output:
- Increasing cyanosis
- Decreased cardiac output leading to cardiovascular collapse

Surgical procedures include a series of 3 staged operations:
- Norwood procedure connects the main pulmonary artery to the aorta, a shunt for pulmonary blood flow, and creates a large atrial septal defect.
- Glenn procedure
- Fontan repair procedure
- Heart transplantation in infancy is preferred in many cases, but the shortage of hearts limits this option

Total anomalous pulmonary venous return

Total anomalous pulmonary venous return is a defect in which the 4 pulmonary veins connect to the right atrium by an anomalous connection rather than the right atrium so there is no direct blood flow to the left side of the heart; however, an atrial septal defect is common and allows for the mixed oxygenated and deoxygenated blood to shunt to the left and enter the aorta. There are 4 different types of anomalies, and in some cases pulmonary vein obstruction. If the pulmonary veins are not obstructed, children may be asymptomatic initially. Symptoms include:
- Heart murmur
- Severe postnatal cyanosis or mild cyanosis
- Dyspnea with grunting and sternal retraction or dyspnea on exertion
- Low oxygen saturation (in the 80s if there is no pulmonary obstruction)
- Cardiomegaly (right-sided hypertrophy)

Surgical repair to attach the pulmonary veins to the left atrium and correct any other defects may be done immediately after birth or delayed for 1 to 2 months.

Transposition of great arteries

Transposition of great arteries is the aorta and pulmonary artery arising from the wrong ventricle (aorta from the right ventricle and pulmonary artery from the left), so there is no connection between pulmonary and systemic circulation with deoxygenated blood being pumped back to the body and the oxygenated blood from the lungs is pumped back to the lungs. Septal defects may also occur, allowing some mixing of blood and the ductus arteriosus allows mixing until it closes. Symptoms vary depending upon whether mixing of blood occurs:
- Mild to severe cyanosis
- Symptoms of congestive heart failure
- Cardiomegaly develops in the weeks after birth
- Heart sounds vary depending upon the severity of the defects

Treatment includes:
- Prostaglandin to keep the ductus arteriosus and foramen ovale open. Balloon atrial septostomy to increase size of foramen ovale
- Surgical repair with cardiopulmonary bypass and aortic cross-clamping to transpose arteries to the normal position ("arterial switch"), as well as repair septal defects and other abnormalities

Truncus arteriosus

Truncus arteriosus is the blood from both ventricles flowing into one large artery with one valve, with more blood flowing to the lower pressure pulmonary arteries than to the body, resulting in low oxygen saturation and hypoxemia. Usually, there is a ventricular septal defect so the blood in the ventricles mixes. Symptoms include:
- Congestive heart failure with pulmonary edema because of increased blood flow to lungs
- Typical symptoms of congestive heart failure
- Cyanosis, especially about the face (mouth and nose)

- Dyspnea, increasing on feeding or exertion
- Poor feeding and failure to thrive.
- Heart murmur
- Increased risk for brain abscess and bacterial endocarditis

Treatment includes:
- Palliative banding of the pulmonary arteries to decrease the flow of blood to the lungs
- Surgical repair with cardiopulmonary bypass includes closing the ventricular defect, utilizing the existing single artery as the aorta by separating the pulmonary arteries from it and creating a conduit between the pulmonary arteries and the right ventricle

Ebstein anomaly

Ebstein anomaly is an abnormality of the tricuspid valve separating the right atrium from the right ventricle with the valve leaflets displaced downward and one adhering to the wall so that there is backflow into the atrium when the ventricle contracts. This usually results in enlargement of the right atrium and congestive heart failure. As pressure increases in the right atrium, it usually forces the foramen ovale to stay open so that the blood is shunted to the left atrium, mixing the deoxygenated blood with oxygenated blood that then leaves through the aorta. Symptoms vary widely depending upon the degree of defect and range from asymptomatic to life-threatening. Ebstein anomaly may occur with other cardiac defects. Many children are not diagnosed until their teens. Symptoms include:
- Cyanosis with low oxygen saturation
- Congestive heart failure
- Palpitations, arrhythmias
- Dyspnea on exertion
- Increased risk for bacterial endocarditis

Treatment includes:
- ACE inhibitors, diuretics, and digoxin
- Surgical repair of abnormalities with valve repair or replacement

ASD

An atrial septal defect (ASD) is an abnormal opening in the septum between the right and left atria. Because the left atrium has higher pressure than the right atrium, some of the oxygenated blood returning from the lungs to the left atrium is shunted back to the right atrium where it is again returned to the lungs, displacing deoxygenated blood. Symptoms may be few, depending upon the degree of the defect, but can include:
- Asymptomatic (some infants).
- Congestive heart failure.
- Heart murmur.
- Increased risk for dysrhythmias and pulmonary vascular obstructive disease over time

Treatment may not be necessary for small defects, but larger defects require closure:
- Open-heart surgical repair may be done.
- Heart catheterization and placing of closure device (Amplatzer) across the atrial septal defect.

Atrioventricular canal defect

Atrioventricular canal defect is often associated with Down syndrome and involves a number of different defects, including openings between the atria and ventricles as well as abnormalities of the valves. In partial defects, there is an opening between the atria and mitral valve regurgitation. In complete defects, there is a large central hole in the heart and only one common valve between the atria and ventricles. The blood may flow freely about the heart, usually from left to right. Extra blood flow to the lungs causes enlargement of the heart. Partial defects may go undiagnosed for 20 years.

Symptoms are as follows:
- Typical congestive heart failure signs:
  o Weakness and fatigue
  o Cough and/or wheezing with production of white or bloody sputum
  o Peripheral edema and ascites
  o Dysrhythmia and tachycardia
- Dyspnea
- Poor appetite
- Failure to thrive, low weight
- Cyanosis of skin and lips

Treatment includes:
- Symptom management as indicated
- Open-heart surgery to patch holes in the septum and valve repair or replacement

Patent ductus arteriosus (PDA)

Ventricular septal defect is an abnormal opening in the septum between the right and left ventricles. If the opening is small, the child may be asymptomatic, but larger openings can result in a left to right shunt because of higher pressure in the left ventricle. This shunting increases over 6 weeks after birth with symptoms becoming more evident, but the defect may close within a few years. Symptoms include:
- Congestive heart failure with peripheral edema
- Tachycardia
- Dyspnea
- Difficulty feeding
- Heart murmur
- Recurrent pulmonary infections
- Increased risk for bacterial endocarditis and pulmonary vascular obstructive disease

Treatment includes:
- Diuretics, such as furosemide, may be used for heart failure
- ACE inhibitor (captopril) to decrease pulmonary hypertension
- Surgical repair includes pulmonary banding or cardiopulmonary bypass repair of the opening with suturing or a patch, depending upon the size

Aortic stenosis

Aortic stenosis is a stricture (narrowing) of the aortic valve that controls the flow of blood from the left ventricle, causing the left ventricular wall to thicken as it increases pressure to overcome the valvular resistance, increasing afterload, and increasing the need for blood supply from the coronary arteries. This condition may result from a birth defect or childhood rheumatic fever and tends to worsen over the years as the heart grows.

Symptoms include:
- Chest pain on exertion and intolerance of exercise
- Heart murmur
- Hypotension on exertion may be associated with sudden fainting
- Sudden death can occur
- Tachycardia with faint pulse
- Poor feeding
- Increased risk for bacterial endocarditis and coronary insufficiency
- Increases mitral regurgitation and secondary pulmonary hypertension

Treatment in children may be done before symptoms develop because of the danger of sudden death:
- Balloon valvuloplasty to dilate valve nonsurgically
- Surgical repair of valve or replacement of valve, depending upon the extent of stricture

Coarctation of the aorta

Coarctation of the aorta is a stricture of the aorta, proximal to the ductus arteriosus intersection. The increased blood pressure caused by the heart attempting to pump the blood past the stricture causes the heart to enlarge and also blood pressure to the head and upper extremities to increase while decreasing blood flow to the lower body and extremities. With severe stricture, symptoms may not occur until the ductus arteriosus closes, causing sudden loss of blood supply to the lower body.   Symptoms include:
- Difference in blood pressure between upper and lower extremities
- Congestive heart failure symptoms in infants
- Headaches, dizziness, and nosebleeds in older children
- Increased risk of hypertension, ruptured aorta, aortic aneurysm, bacterial endocarditis, and brain attack

Treatment includes:
- Prostaglandin (alprostadil) to reopen the ductus arteriosus for infants
- Balloon angioplasty
- Surgical resection and anastomosis or graft replacement (usually at 3 to 5 years of age unless condition is severe). Infants who have surgery may need later repair

Pulmonic stenosis

Pulmonic stenosis is a stricture of the pulmonary blood that controls the flow of blood from the right ventricle to the lungs, resulting in right ventricular hypertrophy as the pressure increases in the right ventricle and decreases pulmonary blood flow. The condition may be symptomatic, asymptomatic, or symptoms may not be evident until the child enters adulthood, depending upon the severity of the defect. Pulmonic stenosis may be associated with a number of other heart defects.

Symptoms include:
- Loud heart murmur
- Congestive heart murmur
- Mild cyanosis
- Cardiomegaly
- Angina
- Dyspnea
- Fainting
- Increased risk of bacterial endocarditis

Treatment includes:
- Balloon valvuloplasty to separate the cusps of the valve for children
- Surgical repair includes the (closed) transventricular valvotomy (Brock) procedure for infants and the cardiopulmonary bypass pulmonary valvotomy for older children

Posterior urethral valves

Posterior urethral valves is a urethral abnormality in males only where urethral valves have narrow slit-like openings that impede urinary flow and allow reverse flow, damaging urinary organs, which swell and become engorged with urine. Thirty percent will develop long-term kidney failure. Diagnosis is by fetal ultrasound, voiding cystourethrogram (VCUG) to evaluate extent of valvular abnormality and other urinary defects, endoscopy to examine inside of urinary tract/take tissue samples, blood tests to assess kidney function, and electrolytes. Symptoms vary, depending upon severity:
- Small chest size with poor lung development and respiratory distress secondary to oligohydramnios (usually the most pressing clinical problem).
- Potter facies secondary to oligohydramnios.
- Limb deformities.
- Abdominal mass secondary to enlarged kidneys, bladder, or ascites.
- Sepsis, metabolic acidosis, and azotemia (increased blood levels of urea and other nitrogenous compounds) may develop.

Medical management includes:
- Supportive care
- Antibiotics
- Electrolytes
- Foley catheter

Surgical management includes urinary diversion (usually closed after valve repair) and endoscopic ablation/resection to examine obstruction and remove valve leaflets.

Persistent cloaca

Persistent cloaca is a condition in females with an imperforate anus and the rectum, vagina, and urethra form a single channel with a rectal fistula attached to the posterior wall of the channel. Diagnosis is made with a physical exam showing a single perineal opening. An abdominal mass (hydrocolpos, distended bladder) may occur. A voiding cystourethrogram (VCUG) will show bladder abnormalities if catheterization is possible. Treatment includes:
- Colostomy: Fecal diversion in neonate prevents fecal material from entering urinary system and causing infection
- Decompression of vagina: Prevents infection and scarring and relieves obstruction of urinary tract
- Posterior sagittal anorectovaginourethroplasty (PSARVUP): (Usually 2 months after colostomy.) Rectum is separated from vagina, vagina is separated from urethra, urethra is reconstructed, vagina is reconstructed, and rectum is reconstructed with anoplasty,
- Postoperative anal dilation: 2 weeks after surgery until final size is reached.
- Cystoscopy/ Vaginoscopy: Checks for urethrovaginal fistula
- Colostomy removal: Anastomosis of colon and rectum and colostomy removed

Ambiguous genitalia
If a neonate has ambiguous genitalia, a complete examination should be performed with ultrasound to determine the gender of the child. In some cases, the child may be intersexed, but surgical sexual assignment/reassignment is now usually delayed until the child expresses a gender preference.

Conditions related to ambiguous genitalia include:
- Microphallus: Less than 2.5 cm often associated with hypospadias
- Clitoromegaly: Rectal exam may help to palpate uterus, which is swollen at birth because of maternal hormones. This may be related to neurofibromatosis
- Congenital adrenal hyperplasia: The fetus was exposed to masculinizing hormones during development. Females often exhibit enlarged clitoris or male-appearing genitalia, partial or complete fusion of the labia, giving the appearance of a scrotum (but without testes)
- Androgen insensitivity syndrome: Genetically male infants cannot respond to androgens and are born with external genitalia that range from typically male to typically female, depending upon the severity of the condition
- Ovotestes: Both male and female genitalia and gonads are present

Epispadias

Epispadias is the urethral orifice in an abnormal position with a widened pubic bone. Epispadias often occurs with bladder exstrophy:
- In boys, the urethra may open on the top (dorsum), the sides, or the complete length of the penis. Boys may have a short, wide penis with abnormal chordee (curvature). It is 3 to 5 times more common in males than females
- In girls, the urethra, with a urethral cleft along its length, usually bifurcates the clitoris and labia but may be in the abdomen

Diagnosis is usually made on fetal ultrasound or at birth on examination. Surgical repair, usually during the first year, may include lengthening of the urethra in males as well as bladder neck reconstruction. Multiple surgical procedures may be required to complete reconstruction for both males and females. Circumcision is delayed in males as the foreskin may be used during the repair. Urinary diversion may be necessary if incontinence cannot be corrected

Hypospadias

Hypospadias occurs in 1 in 250 to 300 live male births. It is a congenital defect where the urethra opens onto the anterior surface of the penis, and not in its usual place at the tip. The urethral opening can be anywhere from the base of the penis to close to the tip on the ventral surface of the penis. Normal urine flow usually exits through this abnormally placed meatus. Hypospadias is classified into three different categories:
- First degree: The opening is on the glans
- Second degree: The opening is on the ventral surface of the shaft of the penis
- Third degree: The opening is on the perineum

No immediate management is required as long as the infant is able to void adequately. Surgical repair is usually performed later. Circumcision is delayed until the surgical repair of the hypospadias is performed because the foreskin may be used during the repair.

UPJ

Ureteropelvic junction (UPJ) obstruction is often discovered during prenatal ultrasounds, and is the most common cause of pediatric hydronephrosis (dilation of the renal pelvis). The most common cause of UPJ in the neonate is the lack of proper canalization of the renal pelvis during embryologic development. The obstruction can be mild or severe and may be asymptomatic in the newborn period. An abdominal mass may be the only sign of a UPJ obstruction with hydronephrosis in the newborn. The UPJ obstruction should be evaluated early with renal ultrasound, voiding cystourethrogram, and a renal scan to determine the degree of obstruction and the need for surgical correction. Another congenital anomaly occurs with UPJ obstruction in approximately 50% of cases, so both kidneys should be evaluated. If the obstruction is severe enough, surgical correction via renal pyeloplasty is performed to prevent renal damage.

Inguinal hernia and hydrocele

A mass in the male infant's scrotum may be an inguinal hernia or hydrocele. During fetal development, the testes migrate from the abdominal cavity into the scrotum through the inguinal canal. The processus vaginalis is a membrane surrounding the testes as they migrate, which normally seals shut and forms a thin band of tissue. When it does not seal properly, it leaves an opening between the abdominal cavity and the scrotum:

- An inguinal hernia is an extension of bowel through the inguinal canal, and possibly into the scrotum, that can be reduced (contents returned to the abdominal cavity) with gentle pressure. Surgical repair is necessary
- A hydrocele occurs when fluid enters the scrotum with the migrating testes. A soft, painless mass will be present that will not reduce (its size remains constant). Unlike a hernia a hydrocele will transilluminate. A communicating hydrocele occurs when a small opening only allows fluid to enter the scrotal sac. This type of hydrocele will fluctuate in size throughout the day and is reducible. This may heal without surgical repair

Bladder exstrophy

Bladder exstrophy is eversion of the posterior wall of the bladder through the anterior wall and through the lower abdominal wall with bladder and urethra exposed, a wide pubic arch, anterior displacement of the anus, renal disorders, and abnormalities of reproductive organs in both males and females. Symptoms include urinary and bowel problems related to specific anomalies. Diagnosis is by physical examination to assess abnormalities. Renal ultrasound is done to determine the number of kidneys and presence of hydroureteronephrosis. Treatment includes:

- First stage:
    - Primary closure of bladder: No ostomy necessary if done within 72 hours of birth. Procedures include ureteral stents and suprapubic urinary drainage
    - Bilateral iliac ostomies: Necessary after 72 hours because pelvic ring is not malleable
    - Epispadias repair: May be done in first or second stage
- Second stage:
    - Epispadias repair: Usually done between 6 and 12 months
- Final stage:
    - Bladder neck reconstruction and reimplantation of ureters
    - Permanent urinary diversion: Required by 10% to 15%

VUR

Vesicoureteral reflux (VUR) is a condition in which urine from the bladder backflows into the ureters or kidneys. Normally, a valve exists at the junction of the ureters and the bladder, but in infants with VUR this valve is defective. Prenatally, VUR may be diagnosed by an ultrasound showing dilated ureters or renal pelvis. Postnatally, an infant with VUR may have an abdominal mass, a urinary tract infection, or pyelonephritis. Nonspecific symptoms, such as respiratory distress, vomiting, failure to thrive, and renal failure may indicate pyelonephritis. VUR is more common in Caucasian children, and runs in families. It is more common in siblings who had VUR or if the parent has a history of VUR. Any infant with a history of a urinary tract infection or pyelonephritis should be evaluated for Vesicoureteral reflux with a VCUG.

Neural tube defects

Neural tube defects (NTD) are a spectrum of congenital disorders involving the meninges covering the spinal cord. The neural tube is the embryonic structure that eventually forms the brain and spinal cord. Mild forms are asymptomatic. Severe cases are incompatible with life. Diagnosis is often made in pregnancy by ultrasound or by an elevated level of alpha-fetoprotein in the mother's serum or the amniotic fluid. Causes are multifactorial, with both genetic and environmental components.

Risk factors for NTD include:
- Poor diet lacking in folic acid.
- Family history of a NTD in a parent or sibling
- Maternal obesity with poorly controlled diabetes
- Maternal use of valproic acid or carbamazepine during pregnancy
- Increasing core temperature 3° to 4°F (2°C) through saunas, hot tubs, or fever

Studies have shown that if the mother's ingests 400 micrograms of folic acid daily before and during pregnancy, it protects the fetus from developing an NTD.

Neural tube defects

The neural tube defects, spina bifida and myelomeningocele, are often used interchangeably, but there is a distinction. Spina bifida is a neural tube defect with an incomplete spinal cord and often missing vertebrae that allow the meninges and spinal cord to protrude through the opening. There are 5 basic types:
- Spina bifida: Defect in which the vertebral column is not closed with varying degrees of herniation through the opening.
- Spina bifida occulta: Failure of the vertebral column to close, but no herniation through the opening so the defect may not be obvious.
- Spina bifida cystica: Defect in closure with external sac-like protrusion with varying degrees of nerve involvement.
- Meningocele: Spina bifida cystica with meningeal sac filled with spinal fluid.
- Myelomeningocele: Spina bifida cystica with meningeal sac containing spinal fluid and part of the spinal cord and nerves.

Myelomeningocele, which involves spina bifida cystica with a meningeal sac containing spinal fluid and part of the spinal cord and nerves, comprises about 75% of the total cases of spina bifida. There are numerous physical manifestations.
- Exposed sac poses the danger of infection and cerebrospinal fluid leakage; surgical repair is usually done within the first 48 hours, although it may be delayed for a few days, especially if the sac is intact.
- Chiari type II malformation comprises hypoplasia of the cerebellum and displacement of the lower brainstem into the upper cervical area, which impairs circulation of spinal fluid. It may result in symptoms of cranial nerve dysfunction (dysphonia, dysphagia) and weakness and lack of coordination of upper extremities.
- Neurogenic bladder is common and may require Credé maneuver for infants and later intermittent clean catheterization.

- Fecal incontinence is common and is controlled as the child gets older with diet and bowel training.

Physical manifestations of myelomeningocele include:
- Musculoskeletal abnormalities depend upon the level of the myelomeningocele and the degree of impairment but often involve the muscle and joints of the lower extremities and sometimes the upper. Dysfunction often increases with the number of shunts. Scoliosis and lumbar lordosis are common. Hip contractures may cause dislocations.
- Paralysis/Paresis may vary considerably and be spastic or flaccid. Many children require wheelchairs for mobility, although some are fitted with braces for assisted ambulation.
- Seizures occur in about a quarter of those affected, sometimes related to shunt malfunction.
- Hydrocephalus is present in about 25% to 35% of infants at birth and 60% to 70% after surgical repair with ventriculoperitoneal shunt. Untreated, the ventricles will dilate and brain damage can occur.
- Tethered spinal cord occurs when the distal end of the spinal cord becomes attached to the bone or site of surgical repair and does not move superiorly with growth, causing increased pain, spasticity, and disability, and requiring surgical repair.

Anencephaly

Anencephaly is a neural tube defect in which the embryological neural tube, which forms the brain and spinal cord, fails to close at the cephalic (head) end, resulting in an infant without most of the brain, skull, or scalp so that the top of the head is open. The eyes bulge foreword. Because the forebrain is missing, the child has no cognitive ability or sensation of pain. A rudimentary brain stem may be present, supporting reflexive breathing and cardiac function, but the child's condition is not compatible with life. Most are born as stillborn and others live a few hours or days. There is no treatment possible other than supportive care until death. The condition is often diagnosed with ultrasound. An ethical dilemma exists about the use of these infants' organs for donation with some authorities believing that viable organs should be harvested before brain death.

Encephalocele

Encephalocele is a neural defect that involves a bony defect and herniation of the brain and/or cerebrospinal fluid through part of the skull in a skin-covered sac. In the United States, most commonly the mass is midline in the occipital and occasionally the frontal area. The encephalocele may be as large as the skull or may look like a small nasal polyp. In many cases, other abnormalities may exist, so thorough examination, including angiography and MRI, are usually required. Often, the part of the brain that herniates is disorganized, so the condition may be associated with cognitive impairment, although in mild cases the child has normal mentation. Surgical repair to place the herniated mass inside the skull and to repair the bony defect is the standard treatment. If the sac is left in place, the skin can erode, resulting in meningitis.

Congenital hip dislocation

Congenital hip dislocation (also known as developmental hip dysplasia because the condition often worsens as the child grows) is hip instability resulting from misalignment of the femoral head and acetabulum. Hip instability may present as dislocation, subluxation, or acetabular dysplasia (abnormal structural development of the joint). Symptoms may not be evident until after the neonatal period and involvement of the left hip is more common than the right. There appears to be a genetic tendency and an association with breech birth. Signs include:

- 3 months or younger: Positive Barlow test (pressing on the knees to apply pressure to the head of the femur when hips are flexed causes posterior subluxation). Positive Ortolani test (hips rotated through range of motion and click heard at abduction as femoral head slips).

Referral to orthopedist is indicated for application of Pavlik harness for infants younger than 3 months.

Metatarsus adductus

Metatarsus adductus ("toeing in") is the most common congenital disorder of the foot, occurring in about 1:1000 births. Metatarsus adductus is a convex curve turning the forefoot inward at the tarsometatarsal joint. Metatarsus adductus occurs equally in males and females and is common among siblings. It is believed the condition may be related to position in the uterus, and it is often associated with oligohydramnios. About 50% have bilateral metatarsus adductus and 10% to 15% have hip dysplasia as well. In most cases, simple stretching exercises are the only needed therapy, and most cases resolve by 3 months. If the curvature is more than 15 degrees, serial casting, changed about 1 time weekly, may be necessary to maintain the foot in the correct position. Braces or special orthopedic shoes may be used after casting is completed.

Talipes equinovarus

Talipes equinovarus (clubfoot) is a congenital abnormality of the foot that involves 3 types of deformities:

- The midfoot is directly inferiorly (equinus)
- The hindfoot turns inward (varus)
- The forefoot adducts toward the heel and then turns superiorly in partial supination

Typically, the foot is small, the Achilles tendon shortened, and the lower leg muscles atrophied. The condition begins during the first trimester, so the foot position is very rigid at birth. Clubfoot occurs in about 1:1000 births with a male to female ratio of 2:1. About 50% of cases are bilateral. Cases vary in severity and some may be associated with other abnormalities, such as myelomeningocele. Diagnosis is often made on ultrasound (16 to 20 weeks) or at birth. The cause is unclear, but there appears to be a genetic component. Treatment is by long leg serial casting (changed every 1 to 2 weeks) begun shortly after birth. In some cases, surgery may be required (at 3 to 12 months) followed by casting and bracing.

Tibial bowing

Tibial bowing is deviation of the tibial diaphysis. There are 3 different types, determined by the direction of the deformity:
- Anterolateral: This type of bowing is associated with neurofibromatosis and may be present at birth or become obvious over time. Treatment is with orthosis from above knee to below ankle. Surgery is not done as it can cause pseudoarthrosis.
- Anteromedial: This type is associated with fibular hemimelia (aplasia or hypoplasia). In the past, amputation was common because of a 3-inch length discrepancy at maturity; however, limb-lengthening procedures are often done now.
- Posteromedial: This type of bowing is associated with a calcaneovalgus deformity (flexible flatfoot). There may be muscle weakness and inequality in limb-length (1 to 5 cm at birth). While angular deformities usually resolve over time, the medial bowing often remains, resulting in problems associated with a shortened limb, so limb-lengthening procedures may be considered later.

Congenital scoliosis

Scoliosis is a lateral (S-shaped) spinal curvature more than 10 degrees. Curvature more than 30 degrees produces marked deformity. The curvature of scoliosis may be structural or compensatory. Congenital scoliosis is increasing because of survival of infants with preterm birth. About 10% of congenital scoliosis relates to abnormalities of the intervertebral/vertebral bodies, affecting the growth of the trunk, most commonly hemivertebra. The male to female ratio is 2.5:1 with about a third of the curvatures at the upper thoracic level with decreasing incidence down the spine (5% at lumbosacral area). Thoracolumbar curvatures carry the worst prognosis. About 20% to 50% of cases have other spinal cord abnormalities, and 30% to 60% of these have other anomalies, such as VATER syndrome. Impairment of pulmonary function is a major complication. Bracing is a successful treatment for less than 10% of cases, but it may be used early to prevent further curvature in preparation for later surgery.

Achondroplasia

Achondroplasia is the most common cause of dwarfism, in which bone growth is inhibited as the result of an abnormal gene on chromosome 4. Achondroplasia can be inherited in an autosomal dominant fashion, but the majority of cases (75% to 80%) occur because of spontaneous mutations. Clinical features of achondroplasia apparent at birth include a long narrow torso with short arms and legs. The proximal segment of the limbs (upper arms and thighs) is disproportionately short. The head is large, with frontal bossing and midface hypoplasia. A small hump (gibbus) may be present in the mid-to-lower back. Mild, generalized hypotonia may be present. Monitor the infant's head size for the development of hydrocephalus. The pediatrician may order a skeletal survey to identify many of skeletal features associated with achondroplasia and to help confirm the diagnosis.

OI

Osteogenesis imperfecta (OI) is a genetic disorder of collagen synthesis that results in brittle, easily fractured bones. OI occurs in 1 in 20,000 live births. Collagen is a major component of bone that gives it both strength and flexibility. Infants with OI either produce defective collagen or deficient amounts of collagen. Four different types of OI have been identified, with symptoms ranging from very mild to lethality in the neonatal period. Common features of OI include:
- Brittle bones that fracture easily (fractures may be present at birth)
- Bowing of long bones
- Discolored, brittle teeth
- Blue sclera
- Skeletal deformities, including scoliosis
- Respiratory difficulties
- Weak muscles

Generally, OI is inherited in a dominant fashion, but a new mutation may cause the disorder in approximately 25% of cases. Parents of children diagnosed with OI must be instructed on correct methods of handling, bathing, and placing their child in the crib to sleep to minimize trauma and the development of fractures.

Care of the High-Risk Infant

Preterm assessment

A preterm infant is born prior to 37 weeks gestational age. In the United States, preterm birth is the most important factor influencing infant mortality; preterm infants account for 75% to 80% of all neonatal morbidity and mortality. Health problems associated with premature birth include:
- Respiratory distress syndrome because of inadequate surfactant production (hyaline membrane disease)
- Hypothermia because of inadequate subcutaneous fat, small amounts of brown fat, and large skin surface area to mass ratio
- Hypoglycemia secondary to poor nutritional intake, poor nutritional stores, and increased glucose consumption associated with sepsis
- Skin trauma or infection secondary to fragile, immature skin
- Periods of apnea because of an immature respiratory center in the brain
- Intraventricular hemorrhage

The original cause of the preterm birth (such as maternal infection) may also play an integral role in the likely health problems associated with prematurity.

Respiratory distress syndrome

Respiratory distress syndrome (formerly hyaline membrane disease) occurs in premature infants and is characterized by immature development of the lungs and inadequate production of surfactant, which results in pulmonary edema, alveolar atelectasis, and injury to tissue. Symptoms include:
- Respiratory distress within hours of birth with progressive decrease in breath sounds. Tachypnea more than > 60/min with increasing crackles.
- Expiratory grunt.
- Nasal flaring.
- Cyanosis.
- Paradoxical respirations.
- Decreased capillary filling time (> 3 to 4 seconds).
- Edema of face and distal extremities (hands, soles of feet).
- Oliguria.
- Tachycardia (> 160 bpm).
- Hypoxemia, respiratory failure.

Laboratory findings are as follows:
- ABGs: Arterial PO_2 < 50 mm Hg, $PCO_2 \geq 50$, pH ≤ 7.25.
- Chest radiograph: Decreased volume, hazy fields, and reticulogranular density.

Complications include:
- Pulmonary air leaks
- Bronchopulmonary dysplasia
- Patent ductus arteriosus
- Hypotension
- Renal failure
- Metabolic acidosis
- Sodium imbalance (hypo or hyper)
- Hypoglycemia
- Hypocalcemia
- Anemia
- Intraventricular hemorrhage
- Seizures
- Retinopathy of prematurity
- Death

Respiratory distress syndrome

Respiratory distress syndrome is often self-limiting as the premature infant begins to produce adequate surfactant within 48 to 72 hours, but more aggressive treatment may be indicated:

- Surfactant replacement therapy:
  - Infants who are 27 to 30 weeks gestation are usually provided prophylactic surfactant replacement therapy after birth per endotracheal tube.
  - Surfactant replacement therapy for those with progressive respiratory distress is administered per inline catheter or 5-Fr. orogastric catheter:
    - Beractant: 4 mL/kg, repeated every 6 hours for 48 hours as needed OR
    - Poractant alfa: 2.5 mL/kg in 2 aliquots initially and 1.25 mg/kg every 12 hours as needed OR
    - Calfactant: 3 mL/kg in 2 aliquots every 12 hours to total of 3 doses.
- Other treatment: Supportive treatment.
  - Supplemental oxygen.
  - CPAP via nasal prongs or endotracheal tube with assisted ventilation for hypoxemia (PaO2 < 50 mm Hg) or hypercapnia (PaCO2 > 60 mm Hg).
  - Manage electrolyte imbalances.
  - Manage fluid balance and provide volume replacement.
  - Dopamine or dobutamine for hypotension.
  - Pulse oximetry.

Heat loss in preterm infants

Preterm infants have not yet developed many of the features that full-term infants use to help protect them from heat loss. The characteristics that make premature infants especially vulnerable to cold stress include:

- Larger surface area to body mass ratio that allows for quicker transfer of body heat to the environment
- Decreased amounts of subcutaneous fat that provides insulation from heat loss
- Decreased amounts of brown fat used for non-shivering thermogenesis
- Immature skin that is not completely keratinized is more permeable to evaporative water and heat loss
- Inability to flex the body to conserve heat
- Limited control of skin blood flow mechanisms that conserve heat

Premature neonate correct positioning

Correct positioning of the premature neonate minimizes outside stimuli and mimics the enclosed and calming environment of the womb, helping with the transition to extrauterine life:
- Place the neonate in a flexed position, with his hands close to midline and near his face.
- Create a nest of blankets or pillows to:
    - Help block out light and noise.
    - Give him the impression of a closed environment.
    - Minimize abnormal molding of the head from prolonged pressure on one side.
- Cover the incubator to further keep out sound and light.
- Place the neonate in the prone position (on his stomach) to help to stabilize the chest wall, improve ventilation, and increase the amount of time an infant is in quiet sleep. However, infants should be placed supine (on the back) most of the time, to decrease the chance of SIDS.

Preterm neonatal stress

Premature neonates have a very limited ability to deal with environmental stressors (light, noise, temperature changes, handling, procedures), but these stressors can affect all neonates. Signs of stress include:
- Color changes, such as mottling or cyanosis
- Episodes of apnea and bradycardia
- Activity changes, such as tremors, twitches, frantic activity, arching, and gaze averting
- Flaccid posture (sagging trunk, extremities and face)
- Easy fatigability

"Time out" recovery period includes the following:
- Stop the activity causing the stress
- Reduce unnecessary stimuli (e.g., lower the lights and postpone nonessential manipulation of the neonate)
- Give the neonate a chance to calm or soothe himself
- Bundle the neonate and place him/her in a comforting, side-lying position with the shoulders drawn forward and the hands brought to midline

Special preterm formulas

Preterm formulas are designed with the special requirements of the premature infant in mind. These infants often have an increased caloric requirement to meet growth expectations. Preterm formulas differ from full-term formulas because they provide:
- 24 kcal/oz as opposed to the 20 kcal/oz found in breast milk and formulas for full-term infants
- Increased levels of protein, vitamins, and minerals, particularly increased amounts of vitamin D, calcium, and phosphorus to prevent osteopenia of prematurity
- Less lactose than term formulas, so they are less likely to cause diarrhea

Breast milk can be "fortified" with the addition of human milk fortifiers (HMF) to achieve the same results. Infants are typically switched to a transitional or cow milk–based formula prior to discharge.

Iron supplementation

The premature infant is especially susceptible to iron deficiency because of the lack of maternal iron transfer during the third trimester and the multiple blood samplings that occur with the extensive monitoring of the premature infant. To minimize the risk of iron deficiency anemia, premature infants fed human milk should be started on iron supplementation once they receive full enteral feeds. Studies have shown that premature infants fed a premature formula have better iron stores when that formula is supplemented with 15 mg/L of iron compared with those receiving formula with 3 mg/L of iron. All formula-fed term infants should receive iron-fortified formulas. Breastfed term infants should be given iron supplementation when they are several months old.

FTT

Failure to thrive (FTT) is a descriptive term for infants who exhibit inadequate growth and development, usually measured by the infant below the 5th percentile for weight (and sometimes height). Failure to thrive may relate to physical causes (such as renal disease or congenital heart disease), psychosocial factors (such as poverty, neglect), or idiopathic factors (unexplained). However, many issues may be involved other than just the parent-child relationship:

- Income: Inability to buy sufficient or nutritional food.
- Health beliefs: Infant subjected to extreme or fad diets (vegan, low fat) without ensuring proper nutrition.
- Lack of education: Inadequate knowledge of proper nutritional requirements for children.
- Stress: Illness, single-family home, divorce, lack of employment, incarceration.
- Psychosocial issues: Postpartum depression, other mental illnesses, or Münchausen syndrome by proxy.
- Resistance to feeding: History of nasogastric feedings, cleft lip/palate, or esophageal atresia.
- Inadequate supply of milk: Poor breastfeeding technique or poor milk supply.

Failure to thrive (FTT) is diagnosed first by identifying neonates at risk because of their evidence of growth failure. Diagnostic measures are:
- Weight/height percentile (5th percentile for weight indicative of FTT).
- Feeding/breastfeeding history: Previous 24 hours and 3- to 5-day period.
- Evaluation of genetic factors: Family history, including heights/weights of parents. Identification of food allergies and food restrictions. Evaluation of feeding/nursing behaviors/practices.
- Lab tests as indicated to check for conditions such as anemia.
- Observation of family interactions, situation.

Management includes:
- Nutritional program to reverse evidence of malnutrition.
- Formula: kcal per day = RDA for age in kcal/kg × ideal weight/actual weight.
- Vitamin and mineral supplements.
- Infants (young): Provide supplements to formula; kcal per ounce of formula should not exceed 24.
- Referrals to social workers, welfare, or child protective services as indicated. Behavior modification related to meal times, eating habits interfering with nutrition. Family therapy as indicated. Family education. Structured supportive environment for feeding.
- Persistence in feeding and elimination of distractions.
- Slow introduction of new foods.

Postterm/postmature infant

Many are normal in size and appearance, but some continue to grow in utero and weigh > 4,000 g. They may exhibit postmaturity syndrome (about 5%), putting the infant at increased risk. Characteristis include:
- Alert appearance (may indicated intrauterine hypoxia)
- Skin: Loose, dry, cracking, parchment-like, lacking lanugo or vernix. May have meconium staining, yellow to green (indicating recent)
- Fingernails: Long (sometimes with meconium staining)
- Scalp hair: Long/thick
- Body: Long, thin (fat layers absent)
- Hypoglycemia from nutritional deprivation
- Hypothermia because of decreased brown fat and liver glycogen
- Meconium aspiration (risk increases with oligohydramnios), increasing risk of impaired gas exchange
- Polycythemia as response to hypoxia, increasing risk of impaired tissue perfusion.
- Seizures resulting from hypoxia
- Cold stress (lack of fat stores)
- Congenital anomalies

Postmaturity syndrome

Postmaturity refers to infants born at more than 43 weeks and exhibiting indications of postmaturity syndrome, putting the infant at high risk of morbidity and mortality, with many deaths occurring during labor. Typically, postmature infants experience decreased placental function, with impaired transport of oxygen and nutrients, so that the infant is prone to develop hypoglycemia and hypoxemia during labor. Symptoms include:
- Hypoglycemia: From inadequate nutrition.
- Meconium aspiration syndrome (MAS): From in utero hypoxia.
- Polycythemia: From increased production of erythrocytes in response to hypoxia.
- Congenital anomalies.
- Seizures: From CNS damage related to hypoxia.
- Cold stress: From inadequate development of subcutaneous fat.

Treatment includes:

- Hypoglycemia: Serial glucose testing and glucose infusions with early feedings, if possible, with close monitoring because asphyxia is common in the first 24 hours.
- Meconium-stained amniotic fluid: Amnioinfusion during labor to dilute meconium and decrease incidence of MAS. Oxygen for respiratory distress.
- Polycythemia: Serial hematocrits with fluid resuscitation and partial exchange transfusion.
- Hypothermia: Radiant warmer.

Hypoglycemia

Hypoglycemia, a drop in blood glucose, occurs as the infant is cut off from the mother's glucose supply. Glucose is the main source of energy for the newborn, yet the glucose regulatory system is not well established. The newborn has a sluggish response to large swings in blood glucose, but levels should stabilize within 4 hours. The newborn's brain relies almost exclusively on glucose for energy, utilizes up to 90% of the glucose supplies, and is very sensitive to hypoglycemia. Normal neonatal values vary:

- Cord blood: 45 to 906 mg/dL.
- Premature infant: 20 to 60 mg/dL.
- Neonate: 30 to 60 mg/dL at birth, 40 to 60 mg/dL at day 1.
- Newborn ≥ day 2: 50 to 80 mg/dL.

Hypoglycemia is blood glucose less than 40 mg/dL. The brain will try to increase blood flow to carry more glucose to the "starving" body, but this increases the chances for a brain bleed. When there is not enough glucose available to feed the body, alternative sources of energy are found, such as lactic acid and ketone bodies; however, burning these elements for fuel leads to a state of metabolic acidosis. Glucose administration is not a benign procedure and complications can arise from its usage.

Acute hypoglycemia

Acute hypoglycemia must be treated by a continuous infusion of glucose because a rebound occurrence of acute hypoglycemia can arise if only a glucose bolus is given. The body will produce more insulin to cover the bolus, and the insulin will then start to use up glucose stores as soon as the bolus stops. To prevent this, a steady infusion should be continued for a time period that is sufficient for the infant's insulin production to stabilize. Most infants with hypoglycemia are asymptomatic. Symptoms can include:

- Central nervous system excitation:
  - Jitteriness,
  - High-pitched cry.
  - Exaggerated Moro reflex.
  - Tremors, seizures.
  - Lethargy.
- General depression:
  - Irregular respirations, apnea.
  - Cyanosis.
  - Sweating.
  - Poor feeding.
  - Temperature instability.

Bedside tests for hypoglycemia with reagent sticks may overestimate hypoglycemia and should be confirmed with a serum level. Hypoglycemic infants are treated with either oral or IV infusion of glucose while awaiting results from the laboratory. If the infant is truly hypoglycemic, the blood glucose test is repeated frequently until the infant displays a stable blood glucose level.

IDM

Infants of diabetic mother (IDM) often present with:
- Birth trauma secondary to cephalopelvic disproportion, including shoulder dislocation
- Hypoglycemia from sudden withdrawal of maternal glucose and elevated insulin in the infant
- Respiratory distress syndrome because elevated insulin inhibits surfactant production
- Polycythemia (excessive red blood cell production) and hyperviscosity because elevated insulin and glucose increase the metabolic rate and oxygen consumption
- Iron deficiency because polycythemia leaches iron from the heart and brain
- Hyperbilirubinemia because of increased red blood cell destruction after birth
- Cardiovascular malformations, such as intraventricular hypertrophy with outflow tract obstruction, transposition of the great arteries, ventral septal defects, and coarctation of the aorta
- Congenital malformations, such as anencephaly, spina bifida, renal agenesis, and duodenal atresia
- Electrolyte abnormalities, such as hypocalcemia and hypomagnesemia
- Macrosomia (greater than 4,000 to 4,500 g) because of increased glucose transfer across the placenta

Heroin

Heroin use by the mother has a profound effect on the fetus and the neonate. Infants with prenatal heroin exposure display symmetric intrauterine growth retardation (IUGR) and are often born prematurely. Sixty to 80% of these infants will undergo neonatal abstinence syndrome (NAS). Heroin has a relatively short half-life and symptoms of NAS typically begin 48 to 72 hours after delivery. Several different body systems are affected by NAS and include:
- CNS dysfunction:
  - High-pitched cry hyperactive. Reflexes increased muscle.
  - Irritability.
  - Tremors.
- GI dysfunction:
  - Poor feeding.
  - Periods of frantic sucking or rooting.
  - Vomiting.
  - Loose or watery stools.
  - Vomiting.

- Miscellaneous signs:
  - Frequent yawning
  - Sneezing multiple times
  - Sweating
  - Fever
  - Tachypnea

Withdrawal symptoms

Fetal exposure to drugs, such as opioids, methadone, cocaine, crack, and other recreational drugs, causes withdrawal symptoms in about 60% of infants. There are many variables, including the type of drug and extent and duration of maternal drug use. For example, children may have withdrawal symptoms within 48 hours for cocaine, heroin, and methamphetamine exposure, but there may be delays of up to 2 to 3 weeks for methadone. Short hospital stays after birth make it imperative that children at risk are identified so they can receive supportive treatment, particularly since they often feed poorly and can quickly become dehydrated and undernourished. Polydrug use makes it difficult to describe a typical profile of symptoms, but they usually include:
- Tremors
- Irritability
- Hypertonicity
- High-pitched crying
- Diarrhea
- Dry skin
- Seizures (in severe cases)

Treatment is supportive. Infants with opiate exposure may be given decreasing doses of opiates, such as morphine elixir, with close monitoring until the child is weaned off of the medication.

Intrauterine drug exposure

Managing symptoms of intrauterine drug exposure:
- High-pitched crying:
  - Keep room quiet with low light.
  - Swaddle the infant securely in a flexed position with the arms close to the body. Hold infant close to body. Rock swaddled infant slowly and rhythmically. Walk with swaddled infant held close.
  - Offer pacifier, possibly with sugar solution if acceptable.
  - Give a warm bath.
  - Play soft music.
  - Placing the infant in a dark room with no stimulation at all for a period of time may be effective if other methods fail.
- Inability to sleep:
  - Decrease environmental stimuli/maintain quiet
  - Waterbed or sheepskin

Feed frequently in small amounts

- Nasal stuffiness/sneezing:
  o Aspirate nasopharynx as needed
  o Feed slowly and give time for rest between sucking
  o Monitor respirations
- Poor feeding and frantic sucking (fingers, fist):
  o Feed small, frequent amounts with enteral feedings if necessary
  o Daily weight
  o Provide nonnutritive sucking with pacifier to relieve frantic sucking
- Regurgitation:
  o Weigh frequently and monitor fluids and electrolytes.
  o Observe for dehydration and provide IV fluids as needed.
  o Place supine with head elevated after feedings.
- Hypertonicity:
  o Monitor temperature and decrease environmental temperature if infant's temperature > 37.6°C.
  o Change infant's position frequently to avoid pressure sores. Place on sheepskin or waterbed to prevent pressure.
- Diarrhea:
  o Change diaper frequently and cleanse skin with mild soap and water.
  o Apply skin barrier as needed.
  o Expose irritated skin to air.
- Tremor, seizures:
  o Decrease environmental stimuli and handling.
  o Change position frequently.
  o Observe for scratches, blistering, or abrasions.
  o Place on sheepskin or waterbed to reduce friction and pressure.
  o Maintain patent airway and observe for apnea.
  o Monitor for hyperthermia.

FAS

Maternal ingestion of alcohol may result in fetal alcohol syndrome (FAS), a syndrome of birth defects. Despite campaigns to inform the public, women continue to drink during pregnancy, but no safe amount of alcohol ingestion has been determined, and pregnant women should be advised to abstain. FAS includes:
- Facial abnormalities: Hypoplastic (underdeveloped) maxilla, micrognathia (undersized jaw), hypoplastic philtrum (groove beneath the nose), short palpebral fissures (eye slits between upper and lower lids)
- Neurological deficits: May include microcephaly, intellectual disability, motor delay, hearing deficits. Learning disorders may include problems with visual-spatial and verbal learning, attention disorders, delayed reaction times
- Growth retardation: Prenatal growth deficit persists with slow growth after birth.
- Behavioral problems: Irritability and hyperactivity. Poor judgment in behavior may relate to deficit in executive functions

Indication of brain damage without the associated physical abnormalities is referred to as alcohol-related neurodevelopmental disorder (ARND).

Effects of cesarean delivery

Currently, about 30% of deliveries in the United States are by cesarean, with increasing numbers of women asking for elective cesarean delivery rather than vaginal delivery. However, cesarean deliveries pose more risk for the neonates because the lungs are not cleared of fluid as they are during labor and vaginal delivery, and if gestational age has not been accurately determined, iatrogenic prematurity may occur with associated respiratory distress. Even full-term neonates are at increased risk of transient tachypnea of newborn and persistent pulmonary hypertension. Neonates delivered by cesarean delivery typically have low APGAR scores, sometimes related to effects of anesthesia. While uncommon, the infant can also be cut during the incision. After delivery, the neonate's respiratory status must be monitored carefully, especially for the first 24 to 48 hours.

Congenital varicella syndrome

Varicella infection (chickenpox) in the mother can affect the fetus in different ways, depending upon the time of exposure. Congenital varicella syndrome is characterized by many abnormalities, including eye abnormalities (cataracts, microphthalmia, pendular nystagmus, and retinal scarring), skin abnormalities (hypertrophy and cicatrix scarring), malformation of limbs, hypoplasia of digits, retarded growth, microcephalus, abnormalities of the brain and autonomic nervous system, developmental delay, and intellectual disability. Mortality rates are high (50% or less) for those with severe defects:
- First trimester: 1% risk of congenital varicella syndrome
- Weeks 23 to 20: 2% risk of congenital varicella syndrome
- 5 days before delivery to 2 days after delivery: Neonate may develop congenital varicella (20% to 25%)
- 6 to 12 days after delivery: Neonate may contract congenital varicella but, if breastfeeding, the child may receive the mother's antibodies so the disease will be milder

Hepatitis B, C, and E

Routine screening of all pregnant women and all newborns helps to identify those infected with hepatitis B virus (HBV). Infants are routinely immunized at discharge from hospital, at 2 months, and at 6 months of age. In the case of a premature infant, the immunization schedule is started when the infant weighs 2 kg or is 2 months old. If the mother is HBV positive, surface antigen treatment of that infant should include careful bathing (wearing gloves) to remove all maternal blood and body fluids. The infant should also receive an IM injection of the hepatitis B immunoglobulin within 12 hours of birth. This immunoglobulin treatment is up to 95% effective in preventing the development of the disease in the infant. Hepatitis C is rarely transmitted to the fetus, and of those infected about 75% clear the infection by 2 years. Hepatitis E poses the greatest risk to the mother with a mortality of about 20% during pregnancy and increased risk of fetal complications and death.

Toxoplasmosis

Toxoplasmosis, protozoan infection with *Toxoplasma gondii*, affects about 38% of pregnant women, who have antibodies from previous infection. About 1 in 1,000 pregnant women becomes infected during pregnancy, primarily from ingesting undercooked meat or unpasteurized goat's milk, or contacting infected cat feces. Risk to the fetus is greatest if the disease occurs during the first trimester, often causing severe fetal abnormalities, such as microcephaly and hydrocephalus, or miscarriage. However, risk of fetal transmission is greatest during the third trimester, although 70% are born without indications of infection. Mild infection may be manifest by retinochoroiditis at birth (with other symptoms delayed). Severe infection may result in convulsions and coma from CNS abnormalities. Other abnormalities include hepatomegaly, splenomegaly, anemia, jaundice, and deafness. Maternal treatment to reduce risk of transmission to the fetus includes initially spiramycin (rovamycin). Pyrimethamine (*Daraprim*) and sulfonamide are usually given after the 18th week. Some studies indicate treatment does not reduce the rate of mother-infant transmission but reduces the severity of abnormalities.

Group B Streptococcus

Group B streptococcus is the most common neonatal bacterial infection. Many women are asymptomatic carriers. Screening of all pregnant women around 36 weeks of gestation followed by antibiotic treatment of the mother during labor can prevent neonatal infection. A mother needs at least 4 hours' worth of antibiotic treatment for the infant to benefit. If an infant is born and the mother has not received the recommended treatment, the infant will often be treated with IV ampicillin and gentamicin for 10 to 14 days. If treatment is ineffective or impossible, the infant with a GBS infection that manifests in the first 24 hours after birth may develop pneumonia and/or meningitis, respiratory distress, floppiness, poor feeding, tachycardia, shock, and seizures. An infant may be asymptomatic at birth but have late-onset infection occurring at around 7 to 10 days old. Late-onset infections (usually meningitis) are generally more serious than earlier onset, and survivors often have serious damage, such as intellectual disability, quadriplegia, blindness, deafness, uncontrollable seizures, and hydrocephalus.

GBS

Guillain-Barré syndrome (GBS) is an autoimmune disorder of the myelinated motor peripheral nervous system, often triggered by a viral gastroenteritis or Campylobacter jejuni infection. Congenital and neonatal GBS can occur. Diagnosis is by clinical symptoms, nerve conduction studies, and lumbar puncture, which often show increased protein with normal glucose and cell count, although protein may not increase for a week or more. Needle conduction studies typically shows slowing of conduction. Symptoms may not be evident at birth but can include hypotonia with leg and arm weakness on neonatal exam. Muscle stretch reflexes may be absent. Delayed symptoms include sudden onset of acute flaccid paralysis and respiratory distress. Treatment is supportive. Infants should be hospitalized for observation and placed on ventilator support if forced vital capacity is reduced. While there is no definitive treatment, plasma exchange or IV immunoglobulin shorten the duration of symptoms.

Rubella

Women should always be vaccinated for rubella before becoming pregnant, as exposure to the virus has devastating effects on the newborn. The mother may not experience any symptoms of the disease or only mild symptoms such as mild respiratory problems or rash. If the rubella exposure is during the first 4 to 5 months of pregnancy, the consequences for the infant are greater. Infants exposed to this virus in utero can develop a set of symptoms known as congenital rubella syndrome. This syndrome includes all or some of the following signs and symptoms:

- Intrauterine growth retardation (IUGR)
- Deafness
- Cataracts
- Jaundice
- Purpura
- Hepatosplenomegaly
- Microcephaly
- Chronic encephalitis
- Cardiac defects

HIV/AIDS

Most infants infected with HIV/AIDS acquire the infection from their mothers (vertical transmission). The perinatal transmission rate is 30% in untreated HIV-positive mothers, usually acquired during delivery. Neonates are usually asymptomatic but are at risk for prematurity, low birth weight and small for gestational age (SGA). Infants may show failure to thrive, hepatomegaly, interstitial lymphocytic pneumonia, recurrent infections, and CNS abnormalities. Optimal treatment reduces the perinatal transmission rate to as low as 1% to 2%:

- Antiviral therapy during the pregnancy: A reduced viral load in the mother lessens the likelihood of prenatal transmission
- Elective cesarean delivery before the amniotic membranes rupture. Emergency cesarean, rupture of membranes longer than 4 hours, and the need for an episiotomy all increase the likelihood of infection during delivery
- Antiviral medications for the neonate for the first 6 weeks of life. The first dose should be given within the first 6 to 12 hours after delivery
- Avoiding breastfeeding: The risk of HIV transmission with breastfeeding is 0.7% per month of breastfeeding

Neonatal HIV testing

The immunological status of infants with HIV-positive mothers is assessed in a series of tests performed over the first 2 years in order to institute treatment and decrease transmission to 2% or less:

- Birth (24 hours or less): ELISA and rapid tests are used to identify those neonates who test positive at birth. Confirmatory testing is done with the neonate's blood (not cord blood), usually using DNA polymerase chain reaction (PCR), which is about 99% sensitive by 1 month. RNA PCR may be used for some subtypes of HIV infection.

In the United States, testing is based on identifying mothers with HIV. If the mother's status is not known, then some states require mandatory testing of the infant, but laws vary. Based on positive findings, treatment is begun within 24 hours without waiting for confirmatory test results. Breastfeeding is avoided. Subsequent testing is done at 2, 4, 12, and 18 months.

Secret Key #1 - Time is Your Greatest Enemy

Pace Yourself

Wear a watch. At the beginning of the test, check the time (or start a chronometer on your watch to count the minutes), and check the time after every few questions to make sure you are "on schedule."

If you are forced to speed up, do it efficiently. Usually one or more answer choices can be eliminated without too much difficulty. Above all, don't panic. Don't speed up and just begin guessing at random choices. By pacing yourself, and continually monitoring your progress against your watch, you will always know exactly how far ahead or behind you are with your available time. If you find that you are one minute behind on the test, don't skip one question without spending any time on it, just to catch back up. Take 15 fewer seconds on the next four questions, and after four questions you'll have caught back up. Once you catch back up, you can continue working each problem at your normal pace.

Furthermore, don't dwell on the problems that you were rushed on. If a problem was taking up too much time and you made a hurried guess, it must be difficult. The difficult questions are the ones you are most likely to miss anyway, so it isn't a big loss. It is better to end with more time than you need than to run out of time.

Lastly, sometimes it is beneficial to slow down if you are constantly getting ahead of time. You are always more likely to catch a careless mistake by working more slowly than quickly, and among very high-scoring test takers (those who are likely to have lots of time left over), careless errors affect the score more than mastery of material.

Secret Key #2 - Guessing is not Guesswork

You probably know that guessing is a good idea. Unlike other standardized tests, there is no penalty for getting a wrong answer. Even if you have no idea about a question, you still have a 20-25% chance of getting it right.

Most test takers do not understand the impact that proper guessing can have on their score. Unless you score extremely high, guessing will significantly contribute to your final score.

Monkeys Take the Test

What most test takers don't realize is that to insure that 20-25% chance, you have to guess randomly. If you put 20 monkeys in a room to take this test, assuming they answered once per question and behaved themselves, on average they would get 20-25% of the questions correct. Put 20 test takers in the room, and the average will be much lower among guessed questions. Why?

1. The test writers intentionally write deceptive answer choices that "look" right. A test taker has no idea about a question, so he picks the "best looking" answer, which is often wrong. The monkey has no idea what looks good and what doesn't, so it will consistently be right about 20-25% of the time.
2. Test takers will eliminate answer choices from the guessing pool based on a hunch or intuition. Simple but correct answers often get excluded, leaving a 0% chance of being correct. The monkey has no clue, and often gets lucky with the best choice.

This is why the process of elimination endorsed by most test courses is flawed and detrimental to your performance. Test takers don't guess; they make an ignorant stab in the dark that is usually worse than random.

$5 Challenge

Let me introduce one of the most valuable ideas of this course—the $5 challenge:

You only mark your "best guess" if you are willing to bet $5 on it.
You only eliminate choices from guessing if you are willing to bet $5 on it.

Why $5? Five dollars is an amount of money that is small yet not insignificant, and can really add up fast (20 questions could cost you $100). Likewise, each answer choice on one question of the test will have a small impact on your overall score, but it can really add up to a lot of points in the end.

The process of elimination IS valuable. The following shows your chance of guessing it right:

If you eliminate wrong answer choices until only this many remain:	Chance of getting it correct:
1	100%
2	50%
3	33%

However, if you accidentally eliminate the right answer or go on a hunch for an incorrect answer, your chances drop dramatically—to 0%. By guessing among all the answer choices, you are GUARANTEED to have a shot at the right answer.

That's why the $5 test is so valuable. If you give up the advantage and safety of a pure guess, it had better be worth the risk.

What we still haven't covered is how to be sure that whatever guess you make is truly random. Here's the easiest way:

Always pick the first answer choice among those remaining.

Such a technique means that you have decided, **before you see a single test question**, exactly how you are going to guess, and since the order of choices tells you nothing about which one is correct, this guessing technique is perfectly random.

This section is not meant to scare you away from making educated guesses or eliminating choices; you just need to define when a choice is worth eliminating. The $5 test, along with a pre-defined random guessing strategy, is the best way to make sure you reap all of the benefits of guessing.

Secret Key #3 - Practice Smarter, Not Harder

Many test takers delay the test preparation process because they dread the awful amounts of practice time they think necessary to succeed on the test. We have refined an effective method that will take you only a fraction of the time.

There are a number of "obstacles" in the path to success. Among these are answering questions, finishing in time, and mastering test-taking strategies. All must be executed on the day of the test at peak performance, or your score will suffer. The test is a mental marathon that has a large impact on your future.

Just like a marathon runner, it is important to work your way up to the full challenge. So first you just worry about questions, and then time, and finally strategy:

Success Strategy

1. Find a good source for practice tests.
2. If you are willing to make a larger time investment, consider using more than one study guide. Often the different approaches of multiple authors will help you "get" difficult concepts.
3. Take a practice test with no time constraints, with all study helps, "open book." Take your time with questions and focus on applying strategies.
4. Take a practice test with time constraints, with all guides, "open book."
5. Take a final practice test without open material and with time limits.

If you have time to take more practice tests, just repeat step 5. By gradually exposing yourself to the full rigors of the test environment, you will condition your mind to the stress of test day and maximize your success.

Secret Key #4 - Prepare, Don't Procrastinate

Let me state an obvious fact: if you take the test three times, you will probably get three different scores. This is due to the way you feel on test day, the level of preparedness you have, and the version of the test you see. Despite the test writers' claims to the contrary, some versions of the test WILL be easier for you than others.

Since your future depends so much on your score, you should maximize your chances of success. In order to maximize the likelihood of success, you've got to prepare in advance. This means taking practice tests and spending time learning the information and test taking strategies you will need to succeed.

Never go take the actual test as a "practice" test, expecting that you can just take it again if you need to. Take all the practice tests you can on your own, but when you go to take the official test, be prepared, be focused, and do your best the first time!

Secret Key #5 - Test Yourself

Everyone knows that time is money. There is no need to spend too much of your time or too little of your time preparing for the test. You should only spend as much of your precious time preparing as is necessary for you to get the score you need.

Once you have taken a practice test under real conditions of time constraints, then you will know if you are ready for the test or not.

If you have scored extremely high the first time that you take the practice test, then there is not much point in spending countless hours studying. You are already there.

Benchmark your abilities by retaking practice tests and seeing how much you have improved. Once you consistently score high enough to guarantee success, then you are ready.

If you have scored well below where you need, then knuckle down and begin studying in earnest. Check your improvement regularly through the use of practice tests under real conditions. Above all, don't worry, panic, or give up. The key is perseverance!

Then, when you go to take the test, remain confident and remember how well you did on the practice tests. If you can score high enough on a practice test, then you can do the same on the real thing.

General Strategies

The most important thing you can do is to ignore your fears and jump into the test immediately. Do not be overwhelmed by any strange-sounding terms. You have to jump into the test like jumping into a pool—all at once is the easiest way.

Make Predictions

As you read and understand the question, try to guess what the answer will be. Remember that several of the answer choices are wrong, and once you begin reading them, your mind will immediately become cluttered with answer choices designed to throw you off. Your mind is typically the most focused immediately after you have read the question and digested its contents. If you can, try to predict what the correct answer will be. You may be surprised at what you can predict.

Quickly scan the choices and see if your prediction is in the listed answer choices. If it is, then you can be quite confident that you have the right answer. It still won't hurt to check the other answer choices, but most of the time, you've got it!

Answer the Question

It may seem obvious to only pick answer choices that answer the question, but the test writers can create some excellent answer choices that are wrong. Don't pick an answer just because it sounds right, or you believe it to be true. It MUST answer the question. Once you've made your selection, always go back and check it against the question and make sure that you didn't misread the question and that the answer choice does answer the question posed.

Benchmark

After you read the first answer choice, decide if you think it sounds correct or not. If it doesn't, move on to the next answer choice. If it does, mentally mark that answer choice. This doesn't mean that you've definitely selected it as your answer choice, it just means that it's the best you've seen thus far. Go ahead and read the next choice. If the next choice is worse than the one you've already selected, keep going to the next answer choice. If the next choice is better than the choice you've already selected, mentally mark the new answer choice as your best guess.

The first answer choice that you select becomes your standard. Every other answer choice must be benchmarked against that standard. That choice is correct until proven otherwise by another answer choice beating it out. Once you've decided that no other answer choice seems as good, do one final check to ensure that your answer choice answers the question posed.

Valid Information

Don't discount any of the information provided in the question. Every piece of information may be necessary to determine the correct answer. None of the information in the question is there to throw you off (while the answer choices will certainly have information to throw you off). If two seemingly unrelated topics are discussed, don't ignore either. You can be confident there is a relationship, or it wouldn't be included in the question, and you are probably going to have to determine what is that relationship to find the answer.

Avoid "Fact Traps"

Don't get distracted by a choice that is factually true. Your search is for the answer that answers the question. Stay focused and don't fall for an answer that is true but irrelevant. Always go back to the question and make sure you're choosing an answer that actually answers the question and is not just a true statement. An answer can be factually correct, but it MUST answer the question asked. Additionally, two answers can both be seemingly correct, so be sure to read all of the answer choices, and make sure that you get the one that BEST answers the question.

Milk the Question

Some of the questions may throw you completely off. They might deal with a subject you have not been exposed to, or one that you haven't reviewed in years. While your lack of knowledge about the subject will be a hindrance, the question itself can give you many clues that will help you find the correct answer. Read the question carefully and look for clues. Watch particularly for adjectives and nouns describing difficult terms or words that you don't recognize. Regardless of whether you completely understand a word or not, replacing it with a synonym, either provided or one you more familiar with, may help you to understand what the questions are asking. Rather than wracking your mind about specific detailed information concerning a difficult term or word, try to use mental substitutes that are easier to understand.

The Trap of Familiarity

Don't just choose a word because you recognize it. On difficult questions, you may not recognize a number of words in the answer choices. The test writers don't put "make-believe" words on the test, so don't think that just because you only recognize all the words in one answer choice that that answer choice must be correct. If you only recognize words in one answer choice, then focus on that one. Is it correct? Try your best to determine if it is correct. If it is, that's great. If not, eliminate it. Each word and answer choice you eliminate increases your chances of getting the question correct, even if you then have to guess among the unfamiliar choices.

Eliminate Answers

Eliminate choices as soon as you realize they are wrong. But be careful! Make sure you consider all of the possible answer choices. Just because one appears right, doesn't mean that the next one won't be even better! The test writers will usually put more than one good answer choice for every question, so read all of them. Don't worry if you are stuck between two that seem right. By getting down to just two remaining possible choices, your odds are now 50/50. Rather than wasting too much time, play the odds. You are guessing, but guessing wisely because you've been able to knock out some of the answer choices that you know are wrong. If you are eliminating choices and realize that the last answer choice you are left with is also obviously wrong, don't panic. Start over and consider each choice again. There may easily be something that you missed the first time and will realize on the second pass.

Tough Questions

If you are stumped on a problem or it appears too hard or too difficult, don't waste time. Move on! Remember though, if you can quickly check for obviously incorrect answer choices, your chances of guessing correctly are greatly improved. Before you completely give up, at least try to knock out a couple of possible answers. Eliminate what you can and then guess at the remaining answer choices before moving on.

Brainstorm

If you get stuck on a difficult question, spend a few seconds quickly brainstorming. Run through the complete list of possible answer choices. Look at each choice and ask yourself, "Could this answer the question satisfactorily?" Go through each answer choice and consider it independently of the others. By systematically going through all possibilities, you may find something that you would otherwise overlook. Remember though that when you get stuck, it's important to try to keep moving.

Read Carefully

Understand the problem. Read the question and answer choices carefully. Don't miss the question because you misread the terms. You have plenty of time to read each question thoroughly and make sure you understand what is being asked. Yet a happy medium must be attained, so don't waste too much time. You must read carefully, but efficiently.

Face Value

When in doubt, use common sense. Always accept the situation in the problem at face value. Don't read too much into it. These problems will not require you to make huge leaps of logic. The test writers aren't trying to throw you off with a cheap trick. If you have to go beyond creativity and make a leap of logic in order to have an answer choice answer the question, then you should look at the other answer choices. Don't overcomplicate the problem by creating theoretical relationships or explanations that will warp time or space. These are normal problems rooted in reality. It's just that the applicable relationship or explanation may not be readily apparent and you have to figure things out. Use your common sense to interpret anything that isn't clear.

Prefixes

If you're having trouble with a word in the question or answer choices, try dissecting it. Take advantage of every clue that the word might include. Prefixes and suffixes can be a huge help. Usually they allow you to determine a basic meaning. Pre- means before, post- means after, pro - is positive, de- is negative. From these prefixes and suffixes, you can get an idea of the general meaning of the word and try to put it into context. Beware though of any traps. Just because con- is the opposite of pro-, doesn't necessarily mean congress is the opposite of progress!

Hedge Phrases

Watch out for critical hedge phrases, led off with words such as "likely," "may," "can," "sometimes," "often," "almost," "mostly," "usually," "generally," "rarely," and "sometimes." Question writers insert these hedge phrases to cover every possibility. Often an answer choice will be wrong simply because it leaves no room for exception. Unless the situation calls for them, avoid answer choices that have definitive words like "exactly," and "always."

Switchback Words

Stay alert for "switchbacks." These are the words and phrases frequently used to alert you to shifts in thought. The most common switchback word is "but." Others include "although," "however," "nevertheless," "on the other hand," "even though," "while," "in spite of," "despite," and "regardless of."

New Information

Correct answer choices will rarely have completely new information included. Answer choices typically are straightforward reflections of the material asked about and will directly relate to the question. If a new piece of information is included in an answer choice that doesn't even seem to relate to the topic being asked about, then that answer choice is likely incorrect. All of the information needed to answer the question is usually provided for you in the question. You should not have to make guesses that are unsupported or choose answer choices that require unknown information that cannot be reasoned from what is given.

Time Management

On technical questions, don't get lost on the technical terms. Don't spend too much time on any one question. If you don't know what a term means, then odds are you aren't going to get much further since you don't have a dictionary. You should be able to immediately recognize whether or not you know a term. If you don't, work with the other clues that you have—the other answer choices and terms provided—but don't waste too much time trying to figure out a difficult term that you don't know.

Contextual Clues

Look for contextual clues. An answer can be right but not the correct answer. The contextual clues will help you find the answer that is most right and is correct. Understand the context in which a phrase or statement is made. This will help you make important distinctions.

Don't Panic

Panicking will not answer any questions for you; therefore, it isn't helpful. When you first see the question, if your mind goes blank, take a deep breath. Force yourself to mechanically go through the steps of solving the problem using the strategies you've learned.

Pace Yourself

Don't get clock fever. It's easy to be overwhelmed when you're looking at a page full of questions, your mind is full of random thoughts and feeling confused, and the clock is ticking down faster than you would like. Calm down and maintain the pace that you have set for yourself. As long as you are on track by monitoring your pace, you are guaranteed to have enough time for yourself. When you get to the last few minutes of the test, it may seem like you won't have enough time left, but if you only have as many questions as you should have left at that point, then you're right on track!

Answer Selection

The best way to pick an answer choice is to eliminate all of those that are wrong, until only one is left and confirm that is the correct answer. Sometimes though, an answer choice may immediately look right. Be careful! Take a second to make sure that the other choices are not equally obvious. Don't make a hasty mistake. There are only two times that you should stop before checking other answers. First is when you are positive that the answer choice you have selected is correct. Second is when time is almost out and you have to make a quick guess!

Check Your Work

Since you will probably not know every term listed and the answer to every question, it is important that you get credit for the ones that you do know. Don't miss any questions through careless mistakes. If at all possible, try to take a second to look back over your answer selection and make sure you've selected the correct answer choice and haven't made a costly careless mistake (such as marking an answer choice that you didn't mean to mark). The time it takes for this quick double check should more than pay for itself in caught mistakes.

Beware of Directly Quoted Answers

Sometimes an answer choice will repeat word for word a portion of the question or reference section. However, beware of such exact duplication. It may be a trap! More than likely, the correct choice will paraphrase or summarize a point, rather than being exactly the same wording.

Slang

Scientific sounding answers are better than slang ones. An answer choice that begins "To compare the outcomes…" is much more likely to be correct than one that begins "Because some people insisted…"

Extreme Statements

Avoid wild answers that throw out highly controversial ideas that are proclaimed as established fact. An answer choice that states the "process should be used in certain situations, if…" is much more likely to be correct than one that states the "process should be discontinued completely." The first is a calm rational statement and doesn't even make a definitive, uncompromising stance, using a hedge word "if" to provide wiggle room, whereas the second choice is a radical idea and far more extreme.

Answer Choice Families

When you have two or more answer choices that are direct opposites or parallels, one of them is usually the correct answer. For instance, if one answer choice states "x increases" and another answer choice states "x decreases" or "y increases," then those two or three answer choices are very similar in construction and fall into the same family of answer choices. A family of answer choices consists of two or three answer choices, very similar in construction, but often with directly opposite meanings. Usually the correct answer choice will be in that family of answer choices. The "odd man out" or answer choice that doesn't seem to fit the parallel construction of the other answer choices is more likely to be incorrect.

Special Report: How to Overcome Test Anxiety

The very nature of tests caters to some level of anxiety, nervousness, or tension, just as we feel for any important event that occurs in our lives. A little bit of anxiety or nervousness can be a good thing. It helps us with motivation, and makes achievement just that much sweeter. However, too much anxiety can be a problem, especially if it hinders our ability to function and perform.

"Test anxiety," is the term that refers to the emotional reactions that some test-takers experience when faced with a test or exam. Having a fear of testing and exams is based upon a rational fear, since the test-taker's performance can shape the course of an academic career. Nevertheless, experiencing excessive fear of examinations will only interfere with the test-taker's ability to perform and chance to be successful.

There are a large variety of causes that can contribute to the development and sensation of test anxiety. These include, but are not limited to, lack of preparation and worrying about issues surrounding the test.

Lack of Preparation

Lack of preparation can be identified by the following behaviors or situations:

Not scheduling enough time to study, and therefore cramming the night before the test or exam
Managing time poorly, to create the sensation that there is not enough time to do everything
Failing to organize the text information in advance, so that the study material consists of the entire text and not simply the pertinent information
Poor overall studying habits

Worrying, on the other hand, can be related to both the test taker, or many other factors around him/her that will be affected by the results of the test. These include worrying about:

Previous performances on similar exams, or exams in general
How friends and other students are achieving
The negative consequences that will result from a poor grade or failure

There are three primary elements to test anxiety. Physical components, which involve the same typical bodily reactions as those to acute anxiety (to be discussed below). Emotional factors have to do with fear or panic. Mental or cognitive issues concerning attention spans and memory abilities.

Physical Signals

There are many different symptoms of test anxiety, and these are not limited to mental and emotional strain. Frequently there are a range of physical signals that will let a test taker know that he/she is suffering from test anxiety. These bodily changes can include the following:

Perspiring
Sweaty palms
Wet, trembling hands
Nausea
Dry mouth
A knot in the stomach
Headache
Faintness
Muscle tension
Aching shoulders, back and neck
Rapid heart beat
Feeling too hot/cold

To recognize the sensation of test anxiety, a test-taker should monitor him/herself for the following sensations:

The physical distress symptoms as listed above
Emotional sensitivity, expressing emotional feelings such as the need to cry or laugh too much, or a sensation of anger or helplessness
A decreased ability to think, causing the test-taker to blank out or have racing thoughts that are hard to organize or control.

Though most students will feel some level of anxiety when faced with a test or exam, the majority can cope with that anxiety and maintain it at a manageable level. However, those who cannot are faced with a very real and very serious condition, which can and should be controlled for the immeasurable benefit of this sufferer.

Naturally, these sensations lead to negative results for the testing experience. The most common effects of test anxiety have to do with nervousness and mental blocking.

Nervousness

Nervousness can appear in several different levels:

The test-taker's difficulty, or even inability to read and understand the questions on the test
The difficulty or inability to organize thoughts to a coherent form
The difficulty or inability to recall key words and concepts relating to the testing questions (especially essays)
The receipt of poor grades on a test, though the test material was well known by the test taker

Conversely, a person may also experience mental blocking, which involves:

Blanking out on test questions
Only remembering the correct answers to the questions when the test has already finished.

Fortunately for test anxiety sufferers, beating these feelings, to a large degree, has to do with proper preparation. When a test taker has a feeling of preparedness, then anxiety will be dramatically lessened.

The first step to resolving anxiety issues is to distinguish which of the two types of anxiety are being suffered. If the anxiety is a direct result of a lack of preparation, this should be considered a normal reaction, and the anxiety level (as opposed to the test results) shouldn't be anything to worry about. However, if, when adequately prepared, the test-taker still panics, blanks out, or seems to overreact, this is not a fully rational reaction. While this can be considered normal too, there are many ways to combat and overcome these effects.

Remember that anxiety cannot be entirely eliminated, however, there are ways to minimize it, to make the anxiety easier to manage. Preparation is one of the best ways to minimize test anxiety. Therefore the following techniques are wise in order to best fight off any anxiety that may want to build.

To begin with, try to avoid cramming before a test, whenever it is possible. By trying to memorize an entire term's worth of information in one day, you'll be shocking your system, and not giving yourself a very good chance to absorb the information. This is an easy path to anxiety, so for those who suffer from test anxiety, cramming should not even be considered an option.

Instead of cramming, work throughout the semester to combine all of the material which is presented throughout the semester, and work on it gradually as the course goes by, making sure to master the main concepts first, leaving minor details for a week or so before the test.

To study for the upcoming exam, be sure to pose questions that may be on the examination, to gauge the ability to answer them by integrating the ideas from your texts, notes and lectures, as well as any supplementary readings.

If it is truly impossible to cover all of the information that was covered in that particular term, concentrate on the most important portions, that can be covered very well. Learn these concepts as best as possible, so that when the test comes, a goal can be made to use these concepts as presentations of your knowledge.

In addition to study habits, changes in attitude are critical to beating a struggle with test anxiety. In fact, an improvement of the perspective over the entire test-taking experience can actually help a test taker to enjoy studying and therefore improve the overall experience. Be certain not to overemphasize the significance of the grade - know that the result of the test is neither a reflection of self worth, nor is it a measure of intelligence; one grade will not predict a person's future success.
To improve an overall testing outlook, the following steps should be tried:

Keeping in mind that the most reasonable expectation for taking a test is to expect to try to demonstrate as much of what you know as you possibly can.

Reminding ourselves that a test is only one test; this is not the only one, and there will be others.

The thought of thinking of oneself in an irrational, all-or-nothing term should be avoided at all costs.

A reward should be designated for after the test, so there's something to look forward to. Whether it be going to a movie, going out to eat, or simply visiting friends, schedule it in advance, and do it no matter what result is expected on the exam.

Test-takers should also keep in mind that the basics are some of the most important things, even beyond anti-anxiety techniques and studying. Never neglect the basic social, emotional and biological needs, in order to try to absorb information. In order to best achieve, these three factors must be held as just as important as the studying itself.

Study Steps

Remember the following important steps for studying:

Maintain healthy nutrition and exercise habits. Continue both your recreational activities and social pass times. These both contribute to your physical and emotional well being.

Be certain to get a good amount of sleep, especially the night before the test, because when you're overtired you are not able to perform to the best of your best ability.

Keep the studying pace to a moderate level by taking breaks when they are needed, and varying the work whenever possible, to keep the mind fresh instead of getting bored. When enough studying has been done that all the material that can be learned has been learned, and the test taker is prepared for the test, stop studying and do something relaxing such as listening to music, watching a movie, or taking a warm bubble bath.

There are also many other techniques to minimize the uneasiness or apprehension that is experienced along with test anxiety before, during, or even after the examination. In fact, there are a great deal of things that can be done to stop anxiety from interfering with lifestyle and performance. Again, remember that anxiety will not be eliminated entirely, and it shouldn't be. Otherwise that "up" feeling for exams would not exist, and most of us depend on that sensation to perform better than usual. However, this anxiety has to be at a level that is manageable.

Of course, as we have just discussed, being prepared for the exam is half the battle right away. Attending all classes, finding out what knowledge will be expected on the exam, and knowing the exam schedules are easy steps to lowering anxiety. Keeping up with work will remove the need to cram, and efficient study habits will eliminate wasted time. Studying should be done in an ideal location for concentration, so that it is simple to become interested in the material and give it complete attention. A method such as SQ3R (Survey, Question, Read, Recite, Review) is a wonderful key to follow to make sure that the study habits are as effective as possible, especially in the case of learning from a textbook. Flashcards are great techniques for memorization. Learning to take good notes will mean that notes will be full of useful information, so that less sifting will need to be done to seek out what is pertinent for studying. Reviewing notes after class and then again on occasion will keep the information fresh in the mind. From notes that have been taken summary sheets and outlines can be made for simpler reviewing.

A study group can also be a very motivational and helpful place to study, as there will be a sharing of ideas, all of the minds can work together, to make sure that everyone understands, and the studying will be made more interesting because it will be a social occasion.

Basically, though, as long as the test-taker remains organized and self confident, with efficient study habits, less time will need to be spent studying, and higher grades will be achieved.

To become self confident, there are many useful steps. The first of these is "self talk." It has been shown through extensive research, that self-talk for students who suffer from test anxiety, should be well monitored, in order to make sure that it contributes to self confidence as opposed to sinking the student. Frequently the self talk of test-anxious students is negative or self-defeating, thinking that everyone else is smarter and faster, that they always mess up, and that if they don't do well, they'll fail the entire course. It is important to decreasing anxiety that awareness is made of self talk. Try writing any negative self thoughts and then disputing them with a positive statement instead. Begin self-encouragement as though it was a friend speaking. Repeat positive statements to help reprogram the mind to believing in successes instead of failures.

Helpful Techniques

Other extremely helpful techniques include:

Self-visualization of doing well and reaching goals
While aiming for an "A" level of understanding, don't try to "overprotect" by setting your expectations lower. This will only convince the mind to stop studying in order to meet the lower expectations.
Don't make comparisons with the results or habits of other students. These are individual factors, and different things work for different people, causing different results.
Strive to become an expert in learning what works well, and what can be done in order to improve. Consider collecting this data in a journal.
Create rewards for after studying instead of doing things before studying that will only turn into avoidance behaviors.
Make a practice of relaxing - by using methods such as progressive relaxation, self-hypnosis, guided imagery, etc - in order to make relaxation an automatic sensation.
Work on creating a state of relaxed concentration so that concentrating will take on the focus of the mind, so that none will be wasted on worrying.
Take good care of the physical self by eating well and getting enough sleep.
Plan in time for exercise and stick to this plan.

Beyond these techniques, there are other methods to be used before, during and after the test that will help the test-taker perform well in addition to overcoming anxiety.

Before the exam comes the academic preparation. This involves establishing a study schedule and beginning at least one week before the actual date of the test. By doing this, the anxiety of not having enough time to study for the test will be automatically eliminated. Moreover, this will make the studying a much more effective experience, ensuring that the learning will be an easier process. This relieves much undue pressure on the test-taker.

Summary sheets, note cards, and flash cards with the main concepts and examples of these main concepts should be prepared in advance of the actual studying time. A topic should never be eliminated from this process. By omitting a topic because it isn't expected to be on the test is only setting up the test-taker for anxiety should it actually appear on the exam. Utilize the course syllabus for laying out the topics that should be studied. Carefully go over the notes that were made in class, paying special attention to any of the issues that the professor took special care to emphasize while lecturing in class. In the textbooks, use the chapter review, or if possible, the chapter tests, to begin your review.

It may even be possible to ask the instructor what information will be covered on the exam, or what the format of the exam will be (for example, multiple choice, essay, free form, true-false). Additionally, see if it is possible to find out how many questions will be on the test. If a review sheet or sample test has been offered by the professor, make good use of it, above anything else, for the preparation for the test. Another great resource for getting to know the examination is reviewing tests from previous semesters. Use these tests to review, and aim to achieve a 100% score on each of the possible topics. With a few exceptions, the goal that you set for yourself is the highest one that you will reach.

Take all of the questions that were assigned as homework, and rework them to any other possible course material. The more problems reworked, the more skill and confidence will form as a result. When forming the solution to a problem, write out each of the steps. Don't simply do head work. By doing as many steps on paper as possible, much clarification and therefore confidence will be formed. Do this with as many homework problems as possible, before checking the answers. By checking the answer after each problem, a reinforcement will exist, that will not be on the exam. Study situations should be as exam-like as possible, to prime the test-taker's system for the experience. By waiting to check the answers at the end, a psychological advantage will be formed, to decrease the stress factor.

Another fantastic reason for not cramming is the avoidance of confusion in concepts, especially when it comes to mathematics. 8-10 hours of study will become one hundred percent more effective if it is spread out over a week or at least several days, instead of doing it all in one sitting. Recognize that the human brain requires time in order to assimilate new material, so frequent breaks and a span of study time over several days will be much more beneficial.

Additionally, don't study right up until the point of the exam. Studying should stop a minimum of one hour before the exam begins. This allows the brain to rest and put things in their proper order. This will also provide the time to become as relaxed as possible when going into the examination room. The test-taker will also have time to eat well and eat sensibly. Know that the brain needs food as much as the rest of the body. With enough food and enough sleep, as well as a relaxed attitude, the body and the mind are primed for success.

Avoid any anxious classmates who are talking about the exam. These students only spread anxiety, and are not worth sharing the anxious sentimentalities.

Before the test also involves creating a positive attitude, so mental preparation should also be a point of concentration. There are many keys to creating a positive attitude. Should fears become rushing in, make a visualization of taking the exam, doing well, and seeing an A written on the paper. Write out a list of affirmations that will bring a feeling of confidence, such as "I am doing well in my English class," "I studied well and know my material," "I enjoy this class." Even if the affirmations aren't believed at first, it sends a positive message to the subconscious which will result in an alteration of the overall belief system, which is the system that creates reality.

If a sensation of panic begins, work with the fear and imagine the very worst! Work through the entire scenario of not passing the test, failing the entire course, and dropping out of school, followed by not getting a job, and pushing a shopping cart through the dark alley where you'll live. This will place things into perspective! Then, practice deep breathing and create a visualization of the opposite situation - achieving an "A" on the exam, passing the entire course, receiving the degree at a graduation ceremony.

On the day of the test, there are many things to be done to ensure the best results, as well as the most calm outlook. The following stages are suggested in order to maximize test-taking potential:

Begin the examination day with a moderate breakfast, and avoid any coffee or beverages with caffeine if the test taker is prone to jitters. Even people who are used to managing caffeine can feel jittery or light-headed when it is taken on a test day.
Attempt to do something that is relaxing before the examination begins. As last minute cramming clouds the mastering of overall concepts, it is better to use this time to create a calming outlook.
Be certain to arrive at the test location well in advance, in order to provide time to select a location that is away from doors, windows and other distractions, as well as giving enough time to relax before the test begins.
Keep away from anxiety generating classmates who will upset the sensation of stability and relaxation that is being attempted before the exam.
Should the waiting period before the exam begins cause anxiety, create a self-distraction by reading a light magazine or something else that is relaxing and simple.

During the exam itself, read the entire exam from beginning to end, and find out how much time should be allotted to each individual problem. Once writing the exam, should more time be taken for a problem, it should be abandoned, in order to begin another problem. If there is time at the end, the unfinished problem can always be returned to and completed.

Read the instructions very carefully - twice - so that unpleasant surprises won't follow during or after the exam has ended.

When writing the exam, pretend that the situation is actually simply the completion of homework within a library, or at home. This will assist in forming a relaxed atmosphere, and will allow the brain extra focus for the complex thinking function.

Begin the exam with all of the questions with which the most confidence is felt. This will build the confidence level regarding the entire exam and will begin a quality momentum. This will also create encouragement for trying the problems where uncertainty resides.

Going with the "gut instinct" is always the way to go when solving a problem. Second guessing should be avoided at all costs. Have confidence in the ability to do well.

For essay questions, create an outline in advance that will keep the mind organized and make certain that all of the points are remembered. For multiple choice, read every answer, even if the correct one has been spotted - a better one may exist.

Continue at a pace that is reasonable and not rushed, in order to be able to work carefully. Provide enough time to go over the answers at the end, to check for small errors that can be corrected.

Should a feeling of panic begin, breathe deeply, and think of the feeling of the body releasing sand through its pores. Visualize a calm, peaceful place, and include all of the sights, sounds and sensations of this image. Continue the deep breathing, and take a few minutes to continue this with closed eyes. When all is well again, return to the test.

If a "blanking" occurs for a certain question, skip it and move on to the next question. There will be time to return to the other question later. Get everything done that can be done, first, to guarantee all the grades that can be compiled, and to build all of the confidence possible. Then return to the weaker questions to build the marks from there.

Remember, one's own reality can be created, so as long as the belief is there, success will follow. And remember: anxiety can happen later, right now, there's an exam to be written!

After the examination is complete, whether there is a feeling for a good grade or a bad grade, don't dwell on the exam, and be certain to follow through on the reward that was promised...and enjoy it! Don't dwell on any mistakes that have been made, as there is nothing that can be done at this point anyway.

Additionally, don't begin to study for the next test right away. Do something relaxing for a while, and let the mind relax and prepare itself to begin absorbing information again.

From the results of the exam - both the grade and the entire experience, be certain to learn from what has gone on. Perfect studying habits and work some more on confidence in order to make the next examination experience even better than the last one.

Learn to avoid places where openings occurred for laziness, procrastination and day dreaming.

Use the time between this exam and the next one to better learn to relax, even learning to relax on cue, so that any anxiety can be controlled during the next exam. Learn how to relax the body. Slouch in your chair if that helps. Tighten and then relax all of the different muscle groups, one group at a time, beginning with the feet and then working all the way up to the neck and face. This will ultimately relax the muscles more than they were to begin with. Learn how to breathe deeply and comfortably, and focus on this breathing going in and out as a relaxing thought. With every exhale, repeat the word "relax."

As common as test anxiety is, it is very possible to overcome it. Make yourself one of the test-takers who overcome this frustrating hindrance.

Additional Bonus Material

Due to our efforts to try to keep this book to a manageable length, we've created a link that will give you access to all of your additional bonus material.

Please visit http://www.mometrix.com/bonus948/nurseaceiicare to access the information.